Intermittent Fasting for Beginners

Learn How to Transform Your Body in 30 Days or Less with This Complete Weight Loss Guide for Men and Women

And

The Ketogenic Diet for Beginners

The Complete Guide to the Keto Diet Offering Clarity to Reset and Heal your Body

Table of Contents

Introduction — i
Chapter 1: What is Intermittent Fasting? — 1

- Why fast? — 2
- Why does this kind of eating plan work so well? — 3
- The benefits of going on an intermittent fast — 5
- Types of intermittent fasting — 6

Chapter 2: The Science Behind Fasting — 8

- Alternate Day Fasting and Chronic Disease Prevention Study done in 2007 — 8
- Energy balance and reproductive dysfunction study done in 2013 — 8
- Potential benefits and harms of intermittent fasting study done in 2017 — 9
- A long-term study on the effects of alternate day fasting — 9
- Harvard study shows how intermittent fasting may be the clue to anti-aging — 10

Chapter 3: The Benefits of Short Fasts — 12

- Can help you lose weight — 12
- Following an intermittent fast can help benefit your heart health — 13
- An intermittent fast can help you prevent certain types of cancer — 13
- You will burn off body fat — 13
- Changes the function of hormones, genes, and cells — 14
- You will live longer — 14
- Simplifies life — 14
- It helps you to keep your brain healthier — 15
- It can reduce inflammation throughout the body — 15
- May prevent Alzheimer's — 15
- It can help reduce diabetes and, in some cases, reverse it — 16

Chapter 4: The Different Types of Intermittent Fasts — 17

- The 16/8 Method — 17
- The 5:2 Diet — 18
- The Eat Stop Eat Method — 18
- Alternate Day Fasting — 19
- The Warrior Diet — 19
- Spontaneous Meal Skipping — 19

Chapter 5: What Should I Eat During My Eating Window? — 21
— 21

- During your fasting window — 21
- During your eating window — 22

Can the ketogenic diet make the intermittent fast more effective? ------ 23

Chapter 6: How to Exercise Effectively and Safely While on an Intermittent Fast -- 25

    What's the best exercise to do while fasting? ----------------------------- 26
    What about high intensity interval training? ----------------------------- 26
    Exercising while preserving your muscles -------------------------------- 26
    Allow your body time to adapt to the workout first --------------------- 27
    Stand up and get some walking into your day --------------------------- 27
    Tips to help get the most out of your workouts ------------------------- 28

Chapter 7: Getting the Right Nutrients In – How to Make Sure I Get Enough Nutrition with a Limited Eating Window ---------------------------------- 29
-- 29

Chapter 8: Should I Take Any Supplements to Help with Health and Weight Loss on an Intermittent Fast? -------------------------------------- 31

Chapter 9: Women and Intermittent Fasting – Is It Safe? ------------------ 34

    The female hormones and fasting -- 34
    Why does intermittent fasting affect women more than men? --------- 35
    When should I consider stopping intermittent fasting? ----------------- 35

Chapter 10: The Basics of Meal Planning to Make the Fast Easier --------- 37
-- 37

    The benefits of meal planning -- 37
    Tips for healthy meal planning --- 39

Chapter 11: Easy Ways to Keep Your Hunger at Bay During Your Fasting Window -- 41

    Drink more water and keep yourself hydrated -------------------------- 41
    Slow down your eating --- 41
    Eat plenty of fiber and protein in your meals ---------------------------- 42
    Get enough sleep at night -- 42
    Have a little bit of soup before one of your meals ------------------------ 43
    Light a candle that smells like vanilla ----------------------------------- 43
    Think about the color of your plate ------------------------------------- 43
    Take a picture of your meal -- 43
    Call up a friend --- 43
    Add some greens to your water -- 44
    Do your exercise routine during your fasting window, a few hours before you can eat -- 44

Chapter 12: Setting Up a Support Group to Keep You on Track ----------- 46

    How can a social support system help you lose weight? --------------- 47

Chapter 13: The Other Side of Intermittent Fasting – The Side Effects and Who Shouldn't Go on an Intermittent Fast ---------- 50

    Hunger ---------- 50
    Cravings ---------- 51
    Headaches ---------- 51
    Low energy ---------- 51
    Irritability ---------- 52
    Constipation, bloating, and heartburn ---------- 52
    Feeling cold ---------- 53
    Overeating ---------- 53
    Bathroom trips ---------- 54

Chapter 14: Common Myths About Intermittent Fasting ---------- 55

    Skipping breakfast can make you fat ---------- 55
    Eating frequent meals can help boost up your metabolism ---------- 55
    Small and frequent meals are necessary to lose weight ---------- 56
    The brain needs to always have a supply of glucose to function ---------- 56
    Fasting will put the body into starvation mode ---------- 56
    Intermittent fasting can make me lose muscle ---------- 57
    Intermittent fasting can be bad for your health ---------- 58
    Intermittent fasting will make you overeat ---------- 58

Conclusion ---------- 60
The Ketogenic Diet for Beginners ---------- 61
Introduction ---------- 63

    Keto vs. Atkins ---------- 64
    Keto vs. Paleo ---------- 66

Problems with Modern Diet ---------- 68

    How Diet Has Changed ---------- 68
    Back To Basics ---------- 69
    Look At Your Diet ---------- 70

The Good Parts Of The Keto Diet ---------- 71
Getting Started with Keto ---------- 75

    How Low is Low? ---------- 75
    First Things First ---------- 75
    Macronutrients ---------- 77

The Problems With Keto ---------- 80

    Side Effects ---------- 80
    The Dangers of Keto ---------- 81

Ketosis and How to Reach It — 84

- Reaching Ketosis — 84
- Fuel for the Brain — 84
- How to Reach Optimal Ketosis — 85
- How to Measure Ketosis — 86

Making Keto Work For Everybody — 89

- Keto on a Budget — 89
- Traveling — 90
- Keto While Dining Out — 91
- Keto and the Holidays — 93

Is Keto A Good Fit? — 95

Exercise — 99

- Keto and Cardio — 100
- Weight Lifting and Keto — 101
- Supplementing — 102
- Keto and Exercise in Harmony — 105

Keto While Vegan — 106

- An Overview — 106
- Limiting Carbs — 107
- Simple Alternatives — 108
- Egg Substitutes — 109
- Getting Enough Fat — 110
- Vegan Protein Sources — 111

FAQ — 112
Myths — 119
Good Foods — 124

- What to Eat — 124
- Foods to Avoid — 125

Shopping List — 126
30-Day Meal Plan — 131
Conclusion — 137

Introduction

Congratulations on downloading *Intermittent Fasting for Beginners* and thank you for doing so.

The following chapters will discuss all the steps that you need to get started with intermittent fasting. There are many different diet plans out there that you can choose to go with, but with all the conflicting information, it is hard to know which diet plan is the right one for you. But intermittent fasting is a bit different. Instead of focusing as much on the foods that you get to eat, you will instead focus more on the time periods when you eat, and the times when you will abstain from food. This helps you to limit the number of calories that you eat, improve your metabolism, increase weight loss, and help heal a bunch of health conditions at once.

This guidebook is going to take the time to talk more about intermittent fasting and the steps that you need to take to get started. We start with some of the basics about what intermittent fasting is about and some of the studies and science that prove whether this is a good eating plan or not. We then move on to the different types of intermittent fasts that you can try, the best diet plans to add into this diet, and even how to add in a safe and effective workout program to help you get the best results.

We also spend some time exploring the great health benefits that come with an intermittent fast. While fasting as long been discussed as a thing that is bad for your health, and many people fear starvation mode, you will find that fasting is not as bad as we are used to hearing about. We will devote some time to discussing all the great benefits that come from any type of intermittent fasting that you choose.

From here, we move onto more specifics about how an intermittent fasting will work. We discuss the importance of having a support person there to help you get better results and why a meal plan can make all the difference. Then we move on to some of the special considerations that women need to consider when they go onto an intermittent fast and some of the myths that you may have heard about fasting, but which are actually keeping you away from some of the great benefits that come with fasting.

For years, people have been told advice about dieting that is contrary to what is needed in an intermittent fast. But this is one of the best and most effective ways to cure your metabolism and help you lose weight like nothing before. If you have been considering getting started with intermittent fasting and you aren't sure where to get started, then read through this guidebook and learn exactly what you need to get started!

There are plenty of books on this subject on the market, so thanks again for choosing this one! Every effort was made to ensure it is full of as much useful information as possible. Please enjoy!

Chapter 1: What is Intermittent Fasting?

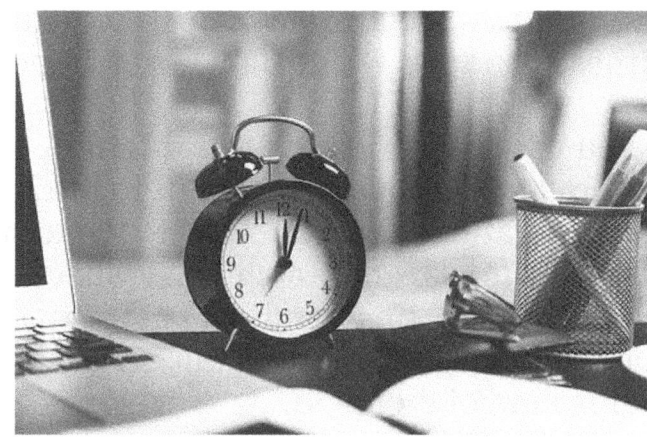

The typical American diet is failing us. There is a lot that is wrong with the way that many Americans choose to eat. Instead of focusing on eating foods that are healthy and wholesome and will provide us the nutrition that we need to stay healthy and disease free, we are eating a lot of processed foods, fast foods, and foods that are full of unnatural ingredients. Instead of listening to our bodies and only eating when we are hungry and need sustenance, we are eating nonstop from the moment we wake up until the moment we go to sleep.

While this is the way that most Americans choose to eat, it is incredibly unhealthy for them. All this eating and all this bad food is causing our bodies to fail. We may be getting plenty of calories, but those calories are empty and don't provide us with the nutrition the body needs to thrive. And all those extra calories are heading straight to our waistline, which is causing a lot of concerning health problems that need to be fixed.

Intermittent fasting is one method that you can use to help fix this problem. It firsts works against the idea that we need to eat five or six meals a day in order to be healthy. Even some popular eating plans ask you to eat that many times in the hopes of keeping your metabolism running fast. But it's not about how many times you eat, but how much you eat that determines the speed of your metabolism. And eating all those times during the day just makes it easier to take in more calories than you need.

With intermittent fasting, you are going to learn how to concentrate your eating periods into smaller increments. This helps you to avoid the issue with eating too much and can make it easier to cut out calories. There are various options that you can choose when it comes to an intermittent fast, including daily fasts, alternate day fasts, and more, so it is really easy to personalize it to fit your needs and your style.

When you are on an intermittent fast, your day is going to be split up into two parts. You will have a fasting period, where you are not allowed to eat anything and can only drink water, coffee, and other drinks that don't have any calories (with the exception of the 5:2 diet where you can eat up to 500 calories on your fasting days). Then there are the eating windows. You can technically eat anything that you want during these times, but these windows will usually be eight hours or less of the day.

While you can eat what you would like on an intermittent fast during your eating window, it is important to remember that if you want to lose weight or really improve your health with this eating plan, you need to make sure that you control your portions, pick out healthy foods, and watch what you eat. You can technically eat whatever you want during that eating window, but if you are going to eat a bunch of bad stuff and junk, then you are going to miss out on the health and wellness benefits that come with this kind of diet plan.

Despite what many people think when they first get started on an intermittent fast, this is actually a pretty easy eating plan that you can enjoy. You don't have to put in a lot of planning ahead of time, unless you want to go on a different diet plan along with this one. And after you go through a few weeks on this eating plan, you are going to enjoy it, be pretty used to it, and feel better with lots more energy than before.

Why fast?

The next question that you may have is why you should consider fasting in the first place. Humans have actually been going through periods of fasting for many years. Sometimes they did this because it was a necessity since they were not able to find any food to eat. Then there were also times that the fasting was done for religious reasons. Religions such as Buddhism, Christianity, and Islam mandate some form of fasting. Also, it is an instinct to fast when you are feeling sick.

Although fasting sometimes has a negative connotation, there is really nothing that is unnatural about fasting. In fact, our bodies are well equipped to handle times when we have to go without eating. There are quite a few processes inside of the body that change when we go on a fast. This helps our bodies to continue functioning during periods of famine.

When we fast, we get a significant reduction in insulin and blood sugar levels, as well as a drastic increase in what is known as the human growth hormone. While this was something that was originally done when food was scarce, it is now used to help people to lose weight. With fasting, burning fat becomes simple, easy, and effective.

Some people decide to go on a fast because it can help their metabolism. This kind of fasting is good for improving various health disorders and diseases. There is also some evidence that shows how intermittent fasting can help you to live longer. Studies show that rodents were able to extend their lifespan with intermittent fasting.

Other research shows that fasting can help protect against various diseases such as Alzheimer's, cancer, type-2 diabetes, and heart disease. And then there are those who choose to go on an intermittent fast because it's convenient for their lifestyle. Fasting can be a really effective life hack. For instance, the fewer meals you have to make, the easier your life will become.

Why does this kind of eating plan work so well?

Another question that a lot of people may have about intermittent fasting is why it actually works so well. Why are you able to simply change around a few of your eating patterns and the times that you eat and see such great results in the process?

Intermittent fasting is when you learn how to schedule your meals so that the body will get the most that it can out of them, and to help you not spend all day eating. Rather than trying to cut out your calories by a bunch and depriving yourself of some of your favorite foods, or diving into a trend diet that never works, intermittent fasting is simple, logical, and can really improve your health without too much work. And the fact that you are able to pick your own approach to intermittent fasting makes it very easy for a lot of people to get on board with it. With intermittent fasting, you don't focus as much on what you eat each day. Rather, you focus more on when you should eat each day.

When you begin with an intermittent fast, it is likely that you will keep your calorie intake similar to what it was before. Some people naturally find that their caloric amount will go down just because they feel full with eating so much during a smaller eating window. So, instead of eating four or five meals a day, you may eat one large meal at 11am and then another one at 6pm, with a fast between 6pm and 11am the next day.

Doing this is one of the methods that you can use with intermittent fasting. It is simple and still allows you to eat. But when you try to put all your calories into just a few meals a day, you are naturally going to eat less, while still feeling full.

Many people have decided to add in intermittent fasting to their daily routines. Individuals like athletes, bodybuilders, and fitness gurus will use it to keep their body fat percentage low and their muscle mass high. It is such a simple strategy and can be adjusted to fit your needs, making it easy to meet all your nutritional needs.

Though the word "fasting" may make alarm the average person, intermittent fasting does not equate to starving yourself. To understand the principals behind successful intermittent fasting, we'll first go over the two body's two states of digestion: the fed state and the fasting state. For three to five hours after eating a meal, your body is in what is known as the "fed state."

During the fed state, your insulin levels increase in order to absorb and digest your food. When your insulin levels are high, it is very difficult for your body to burn fat. Insulin is a hormone produced by the pancreas in order to regulate glucose levels in the bloodstream. Though its purpose is to regulate, insulin is technically a storage hormone. When insulin levels are high, your body is burning your food for energy, rather than your stored fat which is why increased levels of it prevent weight loss.

After the three to five hours are up, your body has finished processing the meal, and you enter the post-absorptive state. The post-absorptive state lasts anywhere from 8 to 12 hours. After this time gap is when your body enters the fasted state. Since your body has completely processed your food by this point, your insulin levels are low, making your stored fat extremely accessible for burning.

In the fasted state, your body has no food left to utilized for energy, so your stored fat is burned instead. Intermittent fasting allows your body to reach an advanced fat burning state that you would normally reach with the average, 'three meals per day' eating pattern. This factor alone is the reason why many people notice rapid results with intermittent fasting without even making changes to their exercise routines, how much they eat, or what they eat. They are simply changing the timing and pattern of their food intake.

It is important to realize that when you first start with a new intermittent fasting program, your body may need a bit of time to get used to this new way of eating. This is a chance to not become discouraged. You may slip up as you get adjusted, but just get back to work and try to get back into the pattern as soon as you can. You will find that any negative self-talk is just going to make things worse and may make you fall back into your old habits for a much longer period of time than you should. Keep working at it, and get through the first few weeks, and intermittent fasting will soon become a normal part of your daily life.

If you have tried out some other diet plans in the past, you may be a bit worried about whether intermittent fasting will work or not. Unlike some of those diet plans, the trends and fads that often seem popular, intermittent fasting is an eating plan that actually works. It is able to work with the natural functioning of your body and you can use this to your advantage to get in better health and lose weight.

You don't have to get too worried about how this intermittent fast is going to work with the starvation mode. The intermittent fast is going to be so effective because it isn't going to let you fast for so long that the body goes into this starvation mode and you stop losing calories and weight. Instead, it is going to make the fast last just long enough that you will actually be able to speed up the metabolism a bit.

With the intermittent fast, you will find that when you go for a few hours without eating, usually no more than 24ish hours at a time, the body is not going to go right into the starvation mode. Rather, it is actually going to speed up through some of the calories that are inside. If you ate the right number of calories for the day, the body is then going to revert to eating up the stored reserves of fat in the body to help fuel it along. So, with this kind of fast, you are avoiding starvation mode and rather turning your body into a machine that is able to eat through more calories than usual without you having to put in more work!

If you are able to pick out the right kind of intermittent fast that you want to follow, stick to it for the long term, and ensure that the foods that you do eat in between your fast are lower in calories, full of healthy nutrition, and good for you, you are going to be pretty amazed at the results that you get from the intermittent fast. Make sure to add in some good weight lifting and cardio exercising, and you will get the results that you want in no time.

As you go through this guidebook, you will soon notice that there is a lot to love about it. You can enjoy a lot of great benefits that will make you feel good, reduce your risk of many chronic illnesses, and can make you lose weight. And you get the benefits of being able to pick the method that works the best for your needs. Whether you like to do a small fast each day and limit your window all the time, or you want to have full day fasts once or twice a week, this type of eating can really make a difference.

Once you get past the idea that an intermittent fast is bad for you or that fasting will put you into starvation mode, you will be able to enjoy all the great things that an intermittent fast can do for you. And once you can get past the first little bit where hunger and cravings can make an intermittent fast hard to do, your body will adjust, and you will fall in love with how easy this type of eating pattern can be.

The benefits of going on an intermittent fast

There are a lot of benefits that come with an intermittent fast lifestyle. All these benefits are the main reason that people like to go on one of these eating plans. And since there are many options in choices when you go on a fast and because you can personalize it to your own needs, an intermittent fast can fit onto any schedule or lifestyle. Some of the benefits that you can enjoy if you choose to go on an intermittent fast include:

- You can lose weight: Many people go on an intermittent fast because it is a great way to help them loose weight. You can easily lose a lot of weight with intermittent fasting by speeding up the metabolism, and naturally eating less with a smaller eating window each day.

- You can cut out belly fat: When your body has to start looking for another source of energy outside of the constant glucose that you usually feed it, it is going to run towards fat. And this often comes in the form of stored body fat. You will see this come in the form of less fat around the belly, and a leaner and trimmer look.

- Reduce your risk of diabetes: When you provide the body with a constant source of glucose, you are putting your body at a higher risk for diabetes. This is because the body will not be able to use all that glucose, and you can develop a resistance to insulin. If you stop providing the body with all this glucose, it gives the body time to heal itself, so you can reduce your risk of diabetes or you can even reverse the diabetes as well.

- Get rid of inflammation throughout the body: An intermittent fast can really help you to reduce inflammation in the body in a natural way. If you combine it with lots of wholesome and healthy foods, you will be able to cut down on the inflammation, and the other health conditions that it causes as well.

- Can give you more energy: Many people report that after a few weeks on an intermittent fast, they start to have more energy than before. The body can burn through the fat stores more efficiently than the glucose that it is used to. While you are going to crave that glucose for a bit at first, you will get used to not having this constant source and will be able to have more energy as you burn through those fat stores instead.

- Helps the brain function better: Once the brain adjusts to knot having that constant source of glucose available, it will start to rely more on the fat stores that are in your body for energy. And since the body can burn through those fat stores efficiently, you get the benefit of a sharper and clearer mind. Think of all the projects you can get done when you are on an intermittent fast.

- Can save money: Since you will start eating fewer meals during the week, you can save a little bit of money. If you do a daily fast, you can cut out a whole seven meals a week, which can help you save your budget. Add in that you aren't going to need as many snacks, and you are going to love how this money can help you and your budget.

There are a lot of different benefits that can come from going on an intermittent fast. These benefits can make a big change in the way that your overall health is and how many chronic diseases you are going to have to face in your own lifetime.

Types of intermittent fasting

There are a few major types of intermittent fasting that you can choose to work with. These fasts can all be effective, and the one that's right for you will depend on your personal preferences, schedule, and lifestyle. Some of the fasting options that you can go with include:

- The 16/8 method: This one will ask you to fast for 16 hours each day and eat during the other 8 hours. So, you may choose to only eat from noon to 8pm or from 10am to 6pm. You can choose whichever eight-hour window that you like.

- Eat-Stop-Eat: Once or twice each week, you will not eat anything from dinner one day until dinner the next day. This gives you a 24-hour fast but still allows you to eat on each of the days that you are fasting.

- The 5:2 diet: You will pick out two days of the week to fast. During those two days, you are only allowed to have up to 500-600 calories each day.

Of course, there are variations of the three that are listed above. For example, some people decide to limit their windows even more and only eat for four hours and fast for twenty on this diet. Most people who go on these fasts will choose to go with the 16/8 method because it's the easiest to stick with and will give you some great results in the process.

Intermittent fasting is simple and effective. It helps you limit the calories that you are consuming and burn more fat and calories than you would with a traditional diet. It may be a bit unusual compared to other forms of eating that you have done before, but it can really make a difference on your overall health and how you feel. As you read through this guidebook, you will soon find that there is so much to love about an intermittent fast and you will wonder why you never tried to use it before.

Chapter 2: The Science Behind Fasting

There are a lot of different studies that can help show how fasting, especially intermittent fasting to help you lose weight and improve your overall health. While conventional wisdom about dieting can't handle intermittent fasting and will go against it quite a bit, this type of eating pattern can make a big difference in weight loss, heart risks, and more. Let's look at some of the research that is behind intermittent fasting:

Alternate Day Fasting and Chronic Disease Prevention Study done in 2007

- The effects that were seen in how well intermittent fasting can work seems to vary between animals and humans. One exception to this is that the animal studies did show a decrease in blood pressure in those animals, but the human trials didn't seem to show this.

- To the date of this study, the affects of alternate day fasting on cancer has only been done on animals. There are many people who believe that these same results would show up in humans who follow fasting as well.

- In terms of how alternate day fasting can help prevent and reduce type 2 diabetes, the results of the data from this study and others have been inconsistent. It may have more to do with the diet plan the individual follows while they are on an intermittent fast. If you continue to eat junk while fasting, type 2 diabetes will not be cured.

Energy balance and reproductive dysfunction study done in 2013

- For this study, rats who were three months old went a period of fasting. They were deprived of any food every other day, going all day long. Then on the non-fasting day, they were fed ad libitum. This went on for 12 weeks.

- During this time, there was a big decrease in mean plasma, luteinizing hormone and testosterone pulse frequency after there was fasting for 48 hours.

- This regimen ended up adversely affecting the reproduction in the rats by changing up the reproductive cycle in the female rats.

- This has been shown in humans as well. While women can also benefit from intermittent fasting, they need to be careful about the number of hours they enter a fasting state. Usually it is recommended that women stick with a fourteen to sixteen hour fast to get the benefits but prevent issues with disrupting their reproductive system.

Potential benefits and harms of intermittent fasting study done in 2017

- There were two studies done on normal and overweight subjects. These individuals reported sustained hunger with this kind of fasting and found that it was difficult for them to maintain daily living activities during restricted days of an alternate day fasting regimen.

- However, in these two studies, when the participants changed to a 16: 8 version of intermittent fasting, these feelings of hunger tended to go away after just a few days.

A long-term study on the effects of alternate day fasting

In the past, one of the biggest issues with intermittent fasting was that there weren't really any long-term studies on it and how it could affect humans. Many of the studies done had been completed with rats and other animals, and any human studies were reviews or only lasted a few weeks. But what about those who decided to use intermittent fasting for the long term want to know if this diet plan is successful or not.

In one study published in JAMA Internal Medicine, people were followed through a whole year. Six months were the individuals trying to lose weight and the other six months were because of a maintenance diet. During the first six months, one third of the subjects could eat what they wanted, one third had their three meals provided each day, which would take up 75 percent of their calorie needs, and the fasting group would alternate between a 500 calorie and a 2500 calorie day.

By the end of this study, both groups kept off about five to six percent of their weight and they all had similar numbers when it came to fasting glucose, insulin resistance, cholesterol, heart rate, and blood pressure. However, the numbers for those in the fasting group may be skewed because 38 percent of the participants dropped out compared to the steady diet losing 29 percent and the control group losing 26 percent. The averages include those who dropped out, so the weight loss may have been different if more people in the intermittent fasters stayed with it longer.

So, this brings up the question about whether intermittent fasting was special or not, or if you should go with a different type of diet. The subjects in this study were metabolically healthy obese women. One of the benefits of intermittent fasting is that it is going to help fix a metabolism that is broken. And the food that these individuals ate was pretty standard and carb heavy. Many people who go on a true intermittent fast will eat lower carb foods, which could help make the results more prominent.

Another thing to note is that this study only looked at one type of intermittent fasting. Many of the studies done on fasting will just work with the 5:2 diet. This one has a little more time between fasts, while other options will have to do a mini fast each day. many claim that the shorter daily fasts are more effective when it comes to losing weight. It may be worth your time to try out the other options for intermittent fasting as well and combine it with a low carb diet to see if that works for you.

When you do go on an intermittent fasting diet, make sure that you also eat a healthy diet and healthy foods as well. You won't be able to lose much weight if you continue to eat junk at the same time. But those who change to a healthier lifestyle and who remain active and get a low carb diet at the same time are the ones who are going to lose more weight with the help of their chosen intermittent fast.

Harvard study shows how intermittent fasting may be the clue to anti-aging

Being able to manipulate the mitochondrial networks that are inside the cells, either by manipulating the genes or restricting your diet, can help you promote health and increase your lifespan. This is according to some new research that comes from the Harvard T.H. Chan School of Public Health.

The study, which was published in Cell Metabolism, sheds some light on how we can work to help prevent aging, or at least slow it down, while also beating out diseases that are related to age. And it could be a solution that is as simple as doing some fasting in our lives to help promote that healthy aging.

Mitochondria, the structures in the cells that will produce energy, exist in networks that are able to change shape based on the demand of energy from the body. Their ability to do this is going to go down with age, but the impact that this can have on cellular function and your metabolism was not understood before. But with this study, researchers are able to show a causal link between dynamic changes in the shapes of your mitochondria and your own longevity.

To test their theories, scientists worked with C.elegans. These only live two weeks, which made it easier for the scientists to study how aging occurs at real time in their labs. The mitochondrial networks that are inside a cell will usually switch between either fragmented or fused states. The researchers found that when they restricted the diet of the worms, or they mimicked a dietary restriction through genetic manipulation, they were able to maintain these mitochondrial networks in a fused, or otherwise known as youthful state. In addition, these youthful networks were able to increase their lifespan by communicating with various organelles to help modulate the metabolism of fat.

While it has long been thought that dietary restrictions and intermittent fasting can help promote health aging, knowing why this all exists is a big step towards helping to harness the benefits and use them for our own needs. These findings from Harvard open up some new avenues in the search for strategies that can reduce a human's likelihood of developing diseases related to age as you get older.

What this means is that when you go on a regular intermittent fast, you may be able to keep the mitochondria in good working order, helping them to remain youthful and helping you to get fewer diseases as you age. The type of diet that works the best for this seems to be the 5:2 diet, but it is possible to see the results with any of the options that are out there for intermittent fasting. The way that you eat can really affect how the genes in our body work, and even how the different parts of the cell behave together, and that can make such a difference in our longevity.

Chapter 3: The Benefits of Short Fasts

Intermittent fasting can help you to fix many different issues throughout the body. Even just a few weeks on an intermittent fast can make a difference in your overall health and if you stick with it for a long time, it can produce even better results. Some of the different benefits that you can receive when you go on an intermittent fast include:

Can help you lose weight

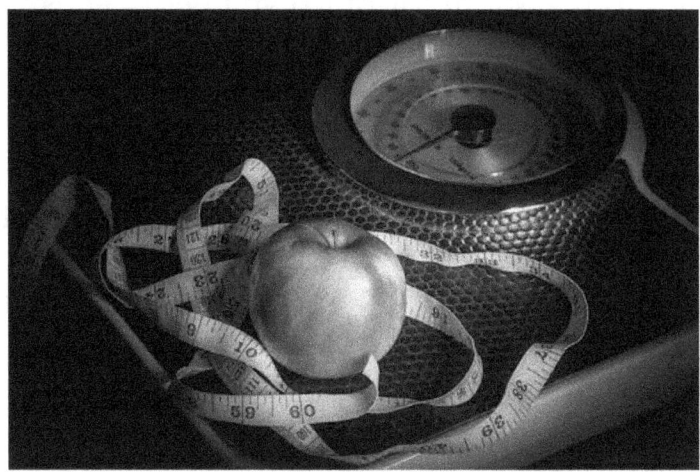

The main reason that a lot of people choose to go on an intermittent fast is to help them lose weight. Over time, if you are careful with your calories and how much you eat, intermittent fasting can force you to eat less without trying as much as before. And when you eat fewer calories, you are able to lose weight. On top of this, intermittent fasting can help enhance the hormone levels and when the body has an increase in the amount of norepinephrine inside, it helps to increase how much body fat is broken down and used for energy.

For this reason, a short term fast can actually help you to increase your metabolic rate up to 14 percent. When your metabolism increases, you will be able to burn even more calories than before. This is one of the neat things about intermittent fasting. It works on both sides of the equation for weight loss. It is going to boost up the metabolic rate, or increases the amount of calories that are going out, and it can reduce the amount of food that you eat, which will reduce the calories that come in.

According to a review in 2014 of scientific literature, it is possible that intermittent fasting will cause a loss in weight of three to eight percent over a period of three to 24 weeks. This is a large amount, especially compared to some of the other diet plans that you may try to go on.

Following an intermittent fast can help benefit your heart health

Currently, heart disease is the biggest killer throughout the world. There are also some health markers, or risk factors, that are often associated with an increase or a decrease in how high your risk for heart disease can be. Intermittent fasting may be the solution that you need to help protect your heart.

Intermittent fasting is tied to many risk factors that can help improve your heart health. This includes blood sugar levels, blood triglycerides, inflammatory markers, LDL cholesterol, total cholesterol, and blood pressure. When these all improve, it is easier to help keep your heart in good working order.

An intermittent fast can help you prevent certain types of cancer

Cancer is a horrible disease that has affected millions of individuals throughout the world. It is characterized by cells growing in an uncontrolled manner. However, intermittent fasting has been shown to make some changes to your metabolism, changes that may be able to reduce your risk of developing cancer over time.

Although most of the studies that have been done on this are from animal studies, the results indicate that it is possible for intermittent fasting to help prevent cancer. There is also some preliminary research that shows how an intermittent fast could help to reduce the bad side effects that come when on a <u>chemotherapy treatment schedule</u>.

You will burn off body fat

In an animal study that was published in "Cell Research" following an intermittent fast for 16 weeks could help prevent obesity. And these early benefits are apparent after only six weeks on the diet. The researchers of this found that intermittent fasting can kickstart your metabolism and can help you burn more fat as the body generates more heat. Intermittent fasting, without reducing calories even, can help provide a therapeutic and preventative approach against a variety of metabolic disorders and even obesity!

For those who have tried to work with other diet plans in the past, being on an intermittent fast can really make a difference. If you do it the right way, it is possible to naturally put the body into the fat burning process. The body will do just fine relying on the stored glycogen in the body, rather than having to keep a steady stream of glucose through the body like our traditional diets require.

It may take some time to get used to. But when you can reduce this dependency on glucose and you let the body rely some more on the stored glycogen and some of the stored fat, and you will be able to see your body burn through more fat than it has on any other diet plan.

Changes the function of hormones, genes, and cells

When you do not eat for some time, several things happen to your body. For example, your body will start initiating processes for cell repair and change some of your hormone levels, which makes stored body fat easier to access. Other changes that can happen in the body include:

- Insulin levels: Your insulin levels will drop by quite a bit, which makes it easier for the body to burn fat.

- Human growth hormone: The blood levels of the growth hormone can greatly increase. Higher levels of this hormone can help build muscle and burn fat.

- Cellular repair: The body will start important cellular repair processes, such as removing all the waste from cells.

- Gene expression: Some beneficial changes occur in several genes that will help you to live longer and protect against disease.

You will live longer

Nothing says that you have been living a healthier lifestyle than longevity. A Harvard study shows how going through an intermittent fast and living with food free periods could manipulate the mitochondria in your cells, resulting in an increased lifespan. As you age, your body is going through a natural decline that is caused by the mitochondria and how they shift. Eating an intermittent fasting diet can help you get healthy aging and a longer lifespan in most individuals.

Simplifies life

While this may not be considered a health benefit like the others, it is still an important one to mention. Many people find that intermittent fasting can make their lives easier. They find that they do not need to focus too much on the calories they are eating, as long as they stay within the hours that they are allowed to eat. They can go a few days a week without having to worry about making a meal. Overall, this diet plan can make your life easier.

When you can cut out some of the work that you need to do during the day and focus on something else, you can end up with less stress in your life. We all know how too much stress can have a negative impact on our health and life. When you can reduce stress, it is much easier to be the healthiest version of yourself.

It helps you to keep your brain healthier

One benefit that everyone seems to agree upon when it comes to intermittent fasting is that it can help promote the healthy functioning of the brain and can even keep away some common neurodegenerative diseases including Parkinson's and Alzheimer's. According to research out of Johns Hopkins School of Medicine, the act of forgoing food can actually challenge your brain. It forces your body and your brain to take measures against diseases.

But how dose this all work? The fasting period will give your body more time to get through the glycogen stores and then makes the body burn off fat instead of sugar. This process is going to produce ketones, which will help boost your energy and banish brain fog. According to the study, packing your meals for the day into eight hours or less, the body will be better equipped to deplete the glycogen stores and then enter into ketosis. This not only helps your body to burn through fat, it can help the brain stay sharp and focused.

It can reduce inflammation throughout the body

For those who are experiencing a lot of inflammation throughout the body on a daily basis, it may be hard to believe that there is a way to help relieve some of the issue. Chronic and long-term inflammation can easily lead to a lot of unwanted belly fat and weight gain, among a whole host of other issues.

This is where intermittent fasting can come into play and help improve your overall health. A study that was done in "Obesity" shows how fasting can produce a very effective anti-inflammatory effect on your system. It works much better than even a high-fat diet is able to do. If you add an intermittent fast in with some foods that are known to be anti-inflammatory, then you are going to see even better results in the process.

May prevent Alzheimer's

Alzheimer's is one of the most common neurodegenerative diseases. There is no cure for Alzheimer's, so your best course of action is to prevent it from happening. One study that was done on rats showed that intermittent fasting might be able to delay the onset of Alzheimer's disease, or at least reduce the severity of it.

Some case reports have shown that a lifestyle alteration that included some daily, or at least frequent, short-term fasts helped to improve the symptoms of Alzheimer's in 9 out of 10 patients. Animal studies also show that this kind of fasting could help to protect against other neurodegenerative diseases, such as Huntington's disease and Parkinson's.

While most of these studies have been done on animals, the results look promising. Intermittent fasting is a trend, and studies on ways it makes your body healthier are relatively new. It will take some time to study the benefits of intermittent fasting.

It can help reduce diabetes and, in some cases, reverse it

Currently, there are more than 29 million people in the United States who are dealing with diabetes. And out of these, at least one in four doesn't know they have the disease. Diabetes is a disease that you can manage with the help of medication, exercise, and the proper diet.

But according to researchers at the University of Southern California, intermittent fasting may be able to help you stop the disease and reverse it. The study notes that following a diet that is like a fast can trigger new pancreatic cells to be produced, and these will go and replace the ones that are dysfunctional in the body. When these new pancreatic cells get into place, they can help you better manage your blood sugar and can make it easier to reverse insulin resistance. If you combine intermittent fasting with a healthy diet, it is easier than ever to manage your diabetes and to help even reverse it in some cases.

These are just a few of the health benefits that you will be able to get when you get started on an intermittent fast. This is really a great option that you can go on to help you lose weight, improve your heart health, and feel better. There haven't been a ton of long-term studies on the effects of intermittent fasting yet, but this is a great diet plan that can give you the results that you want in no time.

Chapter 4: The Different Types of Intermittent Fasts

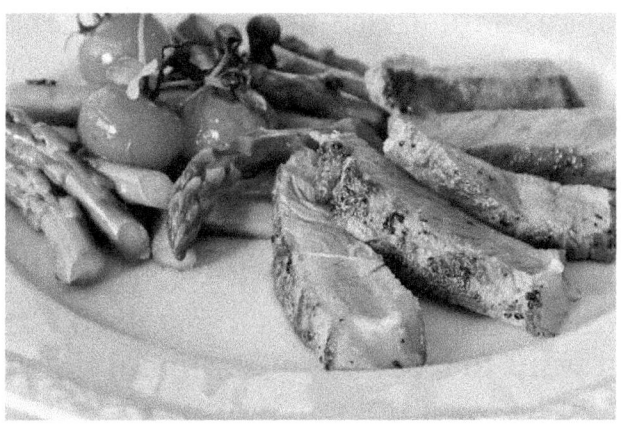

The good thing about an intermittent fast is that you get a choice in the kind you want to go on. There are actually quite a few options that you can choose to go with depending on how long you want to fast, and which one ends up working the best for your schedule. You may find that one is easier for you to implement, and others seem to give you better results than the others. This chapter is going to take a look at some of the different types of intermittent fasts that you can consider using to help you get the amazing results that you want!

The 16/8 Method

A popular method that you can use when it comes to intermittent fasting is the 16/8 method. This is when you will fast each day for a total of 14 to 16 hours, and then you will restrict your eating window for that day to only 8 to 10 hours. When you are in your eating window, you will fit in two or three meals. This helps you to limit the amount of time that you are eating each day, which can naturally cut down on the calories that you consume.

This method is a popular one to follow because it simply could mean not having anything to eat after you finish dinner and then skipping breakfast or moving breakfast back a few hours. So, if you finish your last meal at 6 pm and then don't have a snack or anything after dinner, you could start eating the next day by 10 am, enjoying a late breakfast or an early lunch.

Women who want to go with this type of intermittent fasting should try not to fast for more than sixteen hours. This seems to work better with the hormones and natural rhythm for women and is safer for them to keep up with.

During this type of fast, you are able to drink coffee, water, and other non-caloric beverages to help you reduce the hunger that you feel. And when it comes to the eating window, you need to make sure that you eat a healthy diet rather than a lot of junk or too many calories. This makes it easier for you to maintain the fast and can help you lose weight. In the beginning, you may have some hunger pains as you get used to not being able to eat the second you wake up in the morning, but overall, this is an easy method of intermittent fasting to follow.

The 5:2 Diet

Another popular version of the intermittent fasting diet is known as the 5:2 diet. This one involves the individual eating a normal diet for 5 days of the week. Then they will pick two days of the week where they will keep their calories to between 500 and 600. You can pick the two days that you want to fast on, but try to not have them right by each other, or you may run into troubles with not consuming too much when it's time to eat again.

On these fasting days, you would keep your calories to about 500 for the whole day. Try to get in as many nutrients as possible, but you can also catch up a bit when you get done with the fasting period. Most people split their day into two 250 calorie meals to help them get through this day. but if you are worried about overeating, it may be best to go the day without eating, and then have one 500 calorie meal.

The Eat Stop Eat Method

The eat stop eat method is going to involve doing a 24 hour fast, usually one or two times each week. As long as you don't do the fasting two days in a row. So, you might pick Tuesday and Friday as your fasting days. This method doesn't have to be as difficult as it seems. You could simply stop eating after supper one day and then eat at dinner the next day. This method can ensure that you aren't going to bed hungry each night. Or you can change it up to work with what is best for your schedule. If you want to go from breakfast one day to breakfast the next, or lunch one day to lunch the next, that is fine as well.

During this fast, you are allowed to have coffee, water, and any other non-caloric beverages. But you can't eat any solid food during this time. This can be hard to do, but it can give you some amazing results if you can keep it up. Pick a day when you are going to be pretty busy anyway and would have a lot of trouble getting to a meal, and then this won't be as hard.

If you choose the eat stop eat method to help you lose weight, then you need to make sure that during your eating windows, you eat as normally as you can. Try to eat the same amount of food as you would if you didn't fast. Don't overeat when it is time to start eating again. This helps to even you out to fewer calories through the week and you will lose weight.

Some beginners find that going with the eat stop eat method can be hard. They will feel hungry and they may have trouble making it through the whole day. if you haven't ever done an intermittent fast before, then consider doing one of the smaller fasts first, such as a fast for 16 hours. Get used to this and then move up to the eat stop eat method.

Alternate Day Fasting

With an alternate day fast, you are going to need to fast every other day. You will take one day where you can eat like normal and then the other day needs to be some kind of fast. There are variations on this. Some will ask you not to eat anything during your fasting day, and others will allow you to have around 500 calories during your fasting days.

If you have read any studies on intermittent fasting, including some that are included in this guidebook, the intermittent fasting method they discuss is alternate day fasting. This one can give you a lot of health benefits, but for a beginner, a full day of fasting every other day of the week can be hard. This method is going to leave you feeling hungry several times a week, which can be unpleasant. Starting with a different option can often be the best way to get used to fasting before moving onto this one.

The Warrior Diet

Another option that you can choose is known as the Warrior Diet and this one is often considered the most difficult to follow, simply because the eating window is often small. It can be hard to keep yourself from eating most of the day and it is even harder to get enough nutrients into your day in such a short time period as well.

The Warrior diet is going to involve eating small amounts of vegetables and fruits, raw if possible, during the day. The amount that you take in should only add up to a few hundred calories total. Then you can have one large meal at night. Basically, you are going to be on a fast all day long and then have a feast at night with a four-hour eating window.

The Warrior diet is one of the first popular types of diets that used the idea of intermittent fasting to help. In addition to worrying about such a strict eating window, this diet is going to emphasize food choices that are very similar to being on the Paleo diet. This means that you need to eat foods that are whole, unprocessed, and ones that look like how they do in nature.

Spontaneous Meal Skipping

There are some people who don't want to be on a regular intermittent fast. They don't want to be tied down to something all the time, or maybe they worry about what going on a strict fast would do to their system. But they recognize that it is better for them to listen to their bodies and not just eat non-stop each day. These individuals may choose to go with the process of spontaneous meal skipping or skipping out on meals when it is convenient for them, rather than following a strict schedule.

Any time that you are too busy to cook and sit down to eat, or any time that you just don't feel hungry, you would just skip a meal. It is a myth that people have to get something into their stomachs every few hours or they are going to lose a lot of muscle or they will hit starvation mode. But think about times when you got sick and didn't feel well. You may have gone a few days without eating while you got over an upset stomach, and your metabolism was just fine when you were done.

This is because the human body is set up to handle going longer periods of time when there isn't food. Unlike our modern times, there were often periods when the body would have to go without a lot of food during a famine. Missing a few meals on occasion is not going to be that big of a deal to a body that knows how to prepare for famine.

So, if you feel that you are not hungry at breakfast time one day, you can just skip that meal and eat a dinner and lunch that are healthier. Or, if you are on the road and aren't able to find something that is healthy to eat, go ahead and do a short fast during that time. This isn't the most stringent of intermittent fasts, but it can provide you some of the benefits that you get from the other options. The important thing here is that you must make sure the other meals are healthy and nutrient dense to get the best benefits.

These are just a few of the options that you can choose from when it comes to going on an intermittent fast. There are also variations on each of these that you can choose to work with. All of them can be effective, although the alternate day fasting is the method that is often cited in studies about this type of eating plan. You just need to pick the method that works the best for your lifestyle and the one that helps you reach your goals the best.

If you're finding this book useful please leave a review on Amazon, your feedback is always appreciated!

Chapter 5: What Should I Eat During My Eating Window?

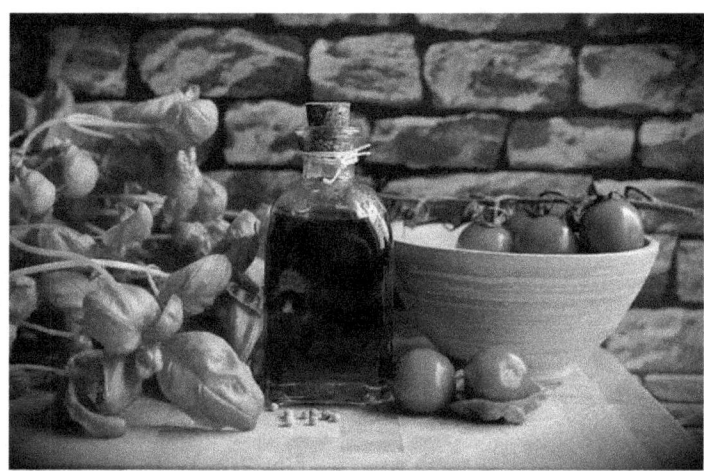

A big question that a lot of people have when they get started on an intermittent fast is what should they eat? They want to make sure that they are getting the most benefits out of this diet plan, without having to feel too deprived. The best thing about an intermittent fast is that you not only get some options with the eating and fasting window, but you also get some choices with the types of food that you want to eat. Some of the suggestions that you can follow to help you do well with eating on an intermittent fast include:

During your fasting window

Most of the options for intermittent fasting are going to follow the same options in what you can eat during your fasting window. During this time, you are not allowed to eat anything. You can have some water, some coffee, or other non-caloric beverages to help you stay hydrated and to keep the hunger away. But you won't eat anything during the fasting time.

This is there to help you get the benefits of your fast. When you go without eating anything, the metabolism will speed up and do a great job burning more calories. It also helps to prevent mindless snacking or eating late at night. You need keep all food away until it is time to enter your eating window.

If you go with the 5:2 diet, there are a few different rules. During your fasting days, you are allowed to have a maximum of 500 calories for that day. This means that you are allowed to eat something, but you need to carefully plan out that day to get the most nutrition possible. Most people split these calories into two meals, and then avoid eating for the rest of the day. There are many great recipes you can rely on to help you get the most out of the few calories you have during that day.

During your eating window

No matter which form of intermittent fasting that you choose to do, you need to make sure that when it is time to eat, you will eat healthy and wholesome foods. Your body is going for long periods of time without food and filling it up with a lot of great nutrition can really help you feel satisfied for longer, improve your health, and lose weight in the process.

A healthy diet can vary for many people. Some choose to go on a diet plan with an intermittent fast to help them get better results. Some just want to eat healthier to help them succeed. If you are simply looking to eat healthier, start with lots of fresh produce. The more variety and color you can get on your plate with each meal, the healthier that meal is. This color helps you to get enough different nutrients into your diet without having to count your macro and micro nutrients each meal.

In addition to eating lots of fresh produce, you need to focus on eating lean cuts of meat. Options like lean ground beef, ground turkey and regular turkey, chicken, and fish can be great options to fill you up and give you the healthy protein and fats that your body needs to stay as healthy as possible. Try to aim for at least a few servings of fish as well. The healthy omega-3 fatty acids and the protein inside the fish can really help fill you up and enhance the fat burning process that intermittent fasting starts.

Healthy grains are allowed on an intermittent fast, as long as you aren't on the ketogenic diet as well. Aim to get whole grains into each meal so that you keep your blood sugar levels steady and to keep you full until the next meal. Be careful about the types of carbs you decide to consume though. Processed and white grains may look the same, but these will turn into glucose in the body and can be stored as body fat when they aren't used up. Whole grains can keep you full for longer, provide you with a ton of great nutrients, and are one of the best ways to complement your meal after a fast.

Whether you choose to add dairy products into your diet will depend on your personal preferences. Some people find that when they go on a fast, they may be more sensitive to dairy products, so they choose to leave these out of their diets. Others find they don't have this sensitivity and having dairy in your diet can be a wonderful addition. Listen to your body and decide if you want to include this into your diet plan or not.

During your intermittent fast, you must be careful about eating a lot of junk and extra calories. If you just resort to eating a lot of processed and junk food after the fast is over, you won't see any weight loss. You need to still come up with a calorie deficit to see results, and while intermittent fasting can help reduce calories and speed up the metabolism on your fasting days, if you catch up with those calories, or surpass them, when you get to eat again, you could even gain weight.

All processed and junk food should be kept down to a minimum. You can eat these on occasion as a treat or a splurge, but they should not be a regular part of your diet plan. And you need to count the calories that you eat during your eating window, or you will still take in too many calories on this fast. If you find that you overindulge too much right after the fast, set up a meal plan that has a lot of healthy nutrition for that first meal, and then scale back on the rest of the meals for the day to keep you in check.

There are a lot of different types of diet plans that you can choose to go with when it comes to intermittent fasting. A lot of people like to stick with something like the ketogenic diet. Those who go on the Warrior diet will focus more on a Paleo style diet. If you are really concerned about your blood pressure, you may consider a DASH diet to help with that. A Mediterranean diet can be another great option to keep you healthy as well. You can pick the diet plan that works the best for you, just make sure you have some plans and can stick with it to see the best results.

Can the ketogenic diet make the intermittent fast more effective?

Many people who go on an intermittent fast to lose weight and improve their health will also consider combining this eating plan with the ketogenic diet as well. There are a lot of great benefits that come with adding these two options together, and when they are combined properly, they can help you to see better results in less time. Some of the benefits of combining a ketogenic diet with your intermittent fast includes:

- You can enter ketosis faster: When your body enters ketosis, it has stopped relying on carbs for energy and instead focuses on using fat as its main source of fuel. This is a more efficient method of energy and will result in you feeling better, clearing out the brain, and not having the big highs or lows that a high carb diet can provide.

- Helps you avoid the side effects from ketosis: If you start with an intermittent fast with your ketosis, you may be able to avoid the keto flu. This is a bit reason that a lot of people consider not going on the ketogenic diet; they are afraid of the horrible flu like symptoms you can get when starting this diet. In addition, following a ketogenic diet can help make your fasting periods easier to manage. Since your body is relying on fat, rather than carbs, you will feel fuller for longer compared to a high carb diet.

- Losing weight faster: Intermittent fasting and the ketogenic diet can really help you to lose a lot of weight quickly. When you combine both, you will be able to lose weight even faster. The smaller eating window can help you to eliminate snacking at night and eating the high fat diet that comes with a keto lifestyle can reduce your appetite and burns fats faster. This can help you lose weight in no time.

- Stabilizes the blood sugars: Someone who is on a regular intermittent fast and who rely on a high carb diet may have issues with spikes in blood sugar. This leads to side effects such as low energy, mood swings, cravings, and brain fog. The ketogenic diet can take away these issues and makes you feel healthier than ever before.

Now, you do not have to go on a ketogenic diet. This is a personal choice, but many people go with this option to enhance the results that you can get from the ketogenic diet. If you do decide to follow this diet plan, there are some different eating rules that you will need to follow to see the results.

About seventy five percent of your calories on this diet plan need to come from healthy fats. You can get these from meat sources, from healthy oils, or from foods like avocados. About twenty percent of your calories should come from healthy sources of protein. Many of the protein sources that you will consume on the ketogenic diet need to have some healthy fats in them too to help you get enough fats in your day.

The last nutrient to concentrate on is the carbs. You are only given five percent of your daily calories to be carbs. And when you choose carbs to consume, they should consist of lots of healthy fruits and vegetables. Many people who want to get into ketosis faster will keep their carb content to under 50 grams a day. This can be hard for many people and you are usually safe sticking with under 100 grams a day if that first limit is too tough.

Eating on the intermittent fast is a personal choice. You can technically go on an intermittent fast and eat anything that you want. But if you choose to consume lots of junk food and extra calories, the intermittent fast is not going to work for you. You can choose to eat a healthy diet that has lots of fresh nutrition, or you can choose a specific diet plan if you want. But the main goal is to stick with your eating window and work to keep the foods that you consume as healthy as possible.

Chapter 6: How to Exercise Effectively and Safely While on an Intermittent Fast

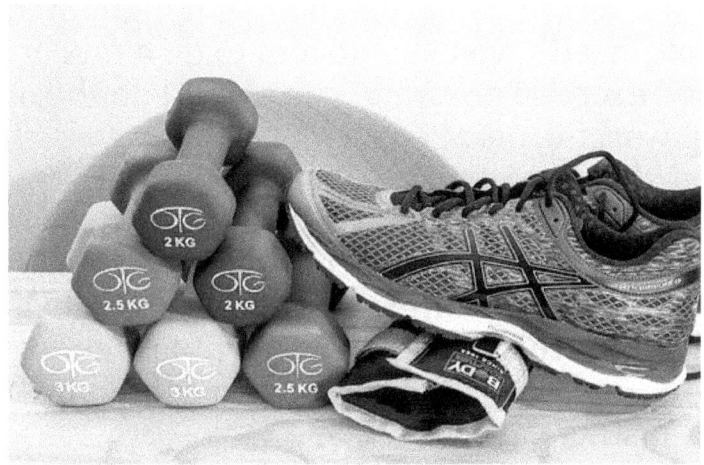

If you are looking to lose weight when you are on an intermittent fast, one of the best things that you can do is start a good exercise program as well. There have been a lot of studies that show how just exercising isn't going to have a big effect on your body weight, but when you combine it together with fasting, it can help boost your weight loss. Any time that you are fasting, your body is going to move on and look for fat for fuel. If you choose to exercise in this state, you are able to burn a lot more fat compared to exercising in a fed state. In addition, exercising while you are fasting can help your body handle carbs in a better way, which can effectively reduce your risk of diabetes.

There are a lot of benefits that come with exercising while on an intermittent fast. Some of these benefits include:

- Exercising while you fast can help improve your performance: Working out before you have breakfast can actually help your performance. The changes that occur are going to improve your fitness faster than anything else.

- Exercising while you fast can help improve how well your muscles repair themselves: A study that was done in mice found that exercise done in a fasted state could actually improve the repair processes of the muscles compared to exercising while you ate.

- Exercise can help stop the hunger pangs: Those who have been on a fast for a long time know that exercising on a fast day can help to get rid of hunger pains. And there is scientific research to confirm this as well.

What's the best exercise to do while fasting?

The benefits of combining fasting with an exercise program will apply to weight training, to moderate and low intensity exercise, and high intensity workouts. To get the most benefits to your health, you should aim to do a mix of all these. However, when it comes to a good exercise program, you should do the one that you enjoy and are most likely to keep working on.

As you get into fasting a bit more, you may find that there are some exercises that are a bit harder to do after a long fast, and this makes them harder to do towards the end of a fast day. High intensity sprinting can be an example of this. The fat that you are going to use for fuel to do this just can't be burnt fast enough to help with this. You can do some jogging and other intense workouts, but you may want to save the sprinting for your non-fasting days.

Options like weight training and walking won't need to use the stored glycogen as much, so they are easier to do. You can add in a little intensity to get the workout up and running better, without worrying about how hard they are on the body or if you will end up too tired to finish them.

What about high intensity interval training?

If you don't feel like spending hours in the gym or outside running, or you want to make sure that you are getting as many health benefits out of your exercise program, then you may want to consider adding in some HIIT to your workout routine.

Research has found that when you do about three rounds of 20 seconds of high intensity exercise three times a week, you can give your body as many benefits as an hour of running on the treadmill. This means you can get the same benefits as running on the treadmill with just a ten to fifteen-minute workout. This can be perfect for those who are just starting on an intermittent fast and just haven't gotten used to the effects of that yet and how much it can wear them out as they get used to the body using up the stored glycogen and fat for energy.

You can choose to do a whole workout based on the idea of HIIT, or you can just incorporate it into your regular workout. For example, if you like to go out and walk for a few miles, add in three or four rounds of higher bursts. You can walk at your normal speed, but then for twenty seconds, start sprinting or running a lot faster. Then go back to your normal speed. This can help you get the workout done faster and can really help improve your fitness without all that much more work.

Exercising while preserving your muscles

Many experts agree that about 80% of the health benefits that you gain from a healthy lifestyle comes from your diet. The rest will come from exercise. This means that you need to focus on eating the right foods if you want to actually lose weight. However, it is important to realize that both exercise and eating well are necessary.

Researchers studied the data from 11 participants who were on the show "The Biggest Loser." The total body fat, total energy expenditure, and the resting metabolic rate of the participants were measured three times. These were measured at the start of the program, after six weeks, and then at 30 weeks. Using a model of the human metabolism, the researchers were able to calculate the impact of diet and exercise changes in resulting in weight loss to see how each one contributed to this goal.

Researchers found that the diet alone was responsible for most of the weight loss. However, only about 65 percent of that weight loss was from body fat. The rest of the reduction in body weight was from lean muscle mass. Exercise alone resulted in fat loss only, along with a slight increase in lean muscle mass.

According to the National Institutes of Health, *"The simulations also suggest that the participants could sustain their weight loss and avoid weight regain by adopting more moderate lifestyle changes – like 20 minutes of vigorous daily exercise and 20 percent calorie restriction – than those demonstrated on the television program."*

Allow your body time to adapt to the workout first

While fasting and exercising can be great things to do together, you don't want to hit the gym too hard when you first get started. For the first few weeks, you should take it slow as you try out fasting and see how your body is going to react to the changes. Until you have been on fasting for a bit, you may not be sure how your body is going to react. If you get through a week of intermittent fasting and you find that you are doing just fine with no problems, then you can go ahead and try adding in some exercise while you fast.

Stand up and get some walking into your day

Walking is a great idea, whether you are working on the intermittent fast or you just want to improve your health. It is good for you, it can help keep you away from food, and it gets you outside. The amount of time that you spend standing up and walking can have a big impact on your weight loss and your overall health. Any standing up and moving around that you do that isn't really exercise, such as walking to get the mail or doing dishes, as non-exercise activity thermogenesis or NEAT.

Overall, NEAT is going to contribute more to how much energy you use during the day than your formal exercise. So, if you are able to increase the levels of NEAT that you have, you can lose weight faster. Those who are on their feet more during the day are often healthier than those who end up spending all day sitting at a desk job.

This doesn't mean that you should give up on your regular workout routine. But it does mean that you should try to get up and move more often during the day. if you work at a desk job, get up for a few minutes every hour to help you circulate the blood and increase your NEAT score.

Tips to help get the most out of your workouts

When you are on an intermittent fast, you are going to quickly notice that things are going to be a bit different on an intermittent fast. Some of the things that you can do to help you get the most out of your workouts during this time will include:

- Start out slowly: Your body has to get used to the new eating pattern, and this can take time. But if you feel like adding in some exercise program after a few weeks, you can do this. Take it slowly and build up to doing more over time. There is no hurry here and even some smaller workouts can make a big difference in how you look and feel while fasting.

- Add in more weights if you feel up to it: Start out with a lower amount of weight and then build up. As soon as you feel like the weight is getting light, you may be able to add some more in. listen to your body and only add on more if it feels right for the situation.

- Fewer reps with more weight is going to help with lean muscles: If you want to build up your lean body mass during this time, remember that fewer reps, but some more weight will really help this happen.

- Remember your warm up and cool down: The warm up and cool down is super important, whether you are in an intermittent fast or not. Spend about five minutes on each to help your body stay healthy and to prevent any injuries or accidents.

- Go slowly and take time off if you need: When you are doing an intermittent fast, you don't want to go crazy with your workouts, no matter what type you are doing. The body needs to adjust to this new way of eating, and you won't be able to hit it quite as hard as you did before. Your energy sources will be a bit lower than before, so just take it easy. If you aren't able to work out each day, or for as hard as you did before, don't be hard on yourself. You will get used to the new routine and be able to gain your strength again.

Chapter 7: Getting the Right Nutrients In – How to Make Sure I Get Enough Nutrition with a Limited Eating Window

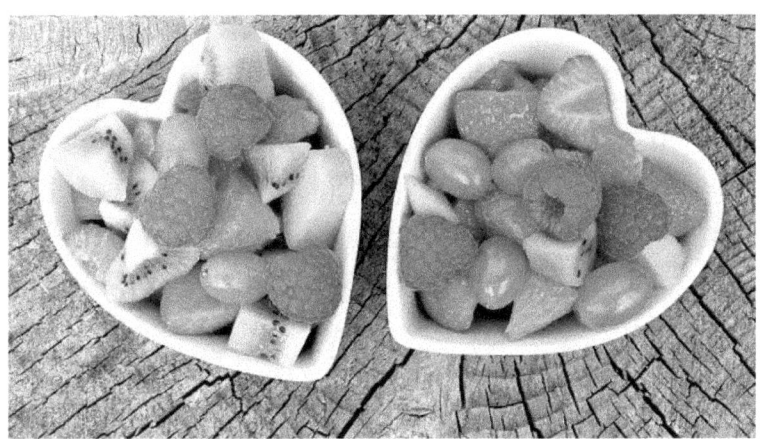

One thing that can be difficult for a lot of people during an intermittent fast is to make sure that they get enough nutrition into their diet when they limit their eating window. The more that you limit your window, the harder it can be to come up with enough nutrition to keep the body healthy. The trick here is to really plan out your days and be mindful of the foods that you are eating during your eating window.

To start, you need to find a calculator or another tool that can help you figure out the number of calories that you should consume every day. this will give you a base number that goes off how many calories you burn just by breathing and being alive, and then adds on for your current height and weight and makes changes based on how active you are during the day. Many of these calculators will also make adjustments to help you figure out a safe caloric amount to go with when you want to lose weight.

Once you have this number, it is time to get planning. You should be able to base your macronutrients from this information as well. You will know exactly how many carbs, fats, and proteins you can have based on your caloric allowance and the diet plan that you want to go on.

Now you need to get to meal planning. We will discuss more about meal planning later on, but this is a great tool to use to help you make sure that you are getting enough nutrients into your day. You can decide how many meals and snacks you want to have during the day and then divide up the nutrients from there. Depending on your eating window, you may want to divide this up between two to three meals. Those on the Warrior diet may even reduce this down to just one meal for the day.

One thing to note here is that many people find themselves very hungry when they get done with a fast, whether they do a daily fast or an alternate day fast. It is best to set up your calories in a way that you can eat more during that first meal after a fast. This helps you to deal with the hunger and cravings you may have right away when the fast ends and won't make you fall off your plan if you just have to have some more. Then, with the other meals and snacks of the day, you can cut down on the calories by just a bit and still stay within your caloric allowance.

When picking out your meal plan, you should include a lot of variety in each meal. This ensures that you will keep your body healthy and will get all the nutrients that you need. When you look at your plate, see all the colors of the rainbow there. This is the easiest way to make sure all the nutrients are covered, without having to go through and find out the nutrients in each item of food. If you are at a loss of which meals to make that will provide your body with a lot of nutrients and will fill you up during your limited eating window, then you can invest in some recipe books and look online to find recipes that have lots of nutrients and will give you the best results from your intermittent fast.

Chapter 8: Should I Take Any Supplements to Help with Health and Weight Loss on an Intermittent Fast?

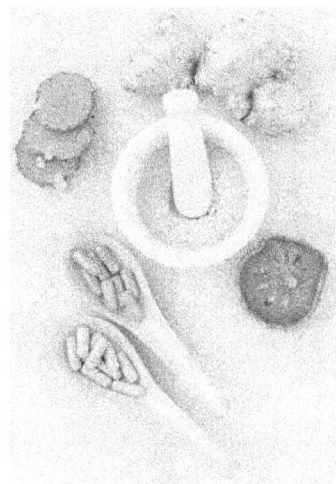

Many of those who are doing an intermittent fast for either weight loss or health reasons wonder whether it is a good idea for them to take a dietary supplement during that time. The worries for this include whether they actually need the nutrition that can come from these supplements and whether this supplement will break their fast and ruin all their efforts.

It is generally recommended that you avoid taking a supplement during your fasting period. And if you eat the proper diet and make sure you aren't missing out on any major food groups during your eating window, you could easily be successful with an intermittent fast without ever having to take a dietary supplement to help you out. However, there are times when taking a supplement, such as during the beginning of the fast as you adjust, may be a good idea to help you out.

One of the benefits that you get with fasting is that while you are doing it, this process is going to put your body in a state that is known as autophagy. This is where the body is cleaning itself out. Most people never give their bodies enough of a break to experience this natural cleansing of the body.

Now, for the most part you should avoid taking any type of supplement when you are in the fasting state to allow the body to go through this cleansing process that you want. But there are some types of supplements that you can take that will help enhance and sometimes speed up this process of autophagy. For example, resveratrol is a supplement that can do this. If you choose to take this supplement, it helps to take it at the beginning of the fast and then again that next morning.

In addition to considering some supplements to enhance the results that you get during the fast, there are also some supplements that you can consider taking when you enter your eating window. These should not be taken during your fasting period because they effectively end the fast, but they can help you give your body the right nutrients when you enter your eating window. Proteins, in the form of whey, and branched chain amino acids are good options and can immediately trigger the body that it is time to end the fast.

Some other supplements that you can take that will help you provide the body with a good amount of nutrition and should be taken when you are in your eating window include fish oils, astaxanthin, probiotics, vitamin D, vitamin K, curcumin, zing, and magnesium. The best times that you can take each of these supplements to get the best benefit out of each one includes:

- Resveratrol: This is a good option that you can take during your fasted state, usually right at the beginning and then again halfway through.

- Magnesium: You can begin your fasted state with a full dose of this. Try to take in this supplement as close to your bedtime as possible to get the best effects.

- Vitamin D: You should start out your eating window with a bit of Vitamin D3.

- Omega-3 fatty acids: You can easily get enough of these from the fish that you should be eating. But if you are taking a supplement, take it at the start of your eating window.

- Vitamin K: You can take this one at the beginning of your eating window. This is an important one to get in because it helps you process calcium in the body.

- IP6: You want to take this one at the end of your eating window, right when you are entering a fast. Or you can take it when you are getting ready for bed and your stomach is empty.

- Glucosamine: You can take this towards the end of your eating window.

- Astaxanthin: This should be taken along with your first meal after you break a fast.

- Nicotinamide: You can take this supplement when you are in the middle of your fast. This supplement is going to help you enhance the effects of the fast.

- Hydroxycitrate: You can also take this one during the middle of your fasting time to help you get more out of the effects.

- Curcumin: This is one that you can take when you are ready to break a fast. Take it with that first meal when it is time to break the fast.

These are important nutrients that you can work with that will either enhance the fasting state or will help keep your body stay healthy while you are on this kind of fast. This is a lot of different supplements though and most people don't want to go through and keep all these on hand. Another option is to pick one or two of these that you want to add into your diet and then add in a multivitamin to pick up the rest.

If you choose to start on a multivitamin, make sure that you choose one that is high quality, and one that has, at a minimum, the nutrients that are listed above. Take it when you break your fast, right at breakfast that day, to get them absorbed into the body as soon as possible.

Taking a supplement is not always a requirement though. You can easily go on an intermittent fast without having to worry about taking these supplements, as long as you pick out a meal plan or a diet that will provide you with these nutrients. But since getting these nutrients can be difficult for those who are first starting on an intermittent fast, or because you want to make sure that you can get the full benefits of a fast, you may want to at least get some supplements to help start out your fast.

Chapter 9: Women and Intermittent Fasting –Is It Safe?

Intermittent fasting is a great eating plan that helps you to reduce your calories and increase your metabolism all in one. There are many ways to do an intermittent fast, which makes it easy for almost everyone to go on one of these fasts. While there are many women who have gone on an intermittent fast and believe that it is one of the best things that they have ever done, there are other women who find that there were serious problems with fasting including lost menstrual periods, metabolic disruption, binge eating, and even early onset menopause. And these could happen to women who are as young as their mid-20s.

So, is it safe for women to go on an intermittent fast? The answer is; it depends. Many women are going to respond to intermittent fasting differently than men, and it often depends on how hard they go into the fast and which type of fasting program they decide to go on. If you plan to start with an intermittent fast as a woman, it is important that you understand how this eating plan can affect you and what precautions you should take to do a fast safely.

The female hormones and fasting

Many people think that intermittent fasting is not a big deal, and that experimenting with it a bit isn't such a big deal. But for some women, small decisions can have a big impact on them. The hormones that are able to regulate some key functions in women, such as ovulation, are going to be incredibly sensitive to the amount of energy that you take in.

In both genders, the hypothalamic pituitary gonadal axis, which is the cooperative functioning of three endocrine glands, can act similar to how you would imagine an air traffic controller. First, your hypothalamus is going to release a hormone that is known as GnRH. This is then going to tell your pituitary gland to release the LH hormone and the FHS hormone.

These two hormones are going to act on the gonads of the individual, which would be either the ovaries or the testes. In women, this means that these hormones are going to trigger the production of progesterone and estrogen, both of which are needed to help release a mature egg and to help support a pregnancy. For men, these hormones are going to trigger the production of testosterone and sperm production.

Because of this chain of reactions that occur at a specific time to make a regular cycle in women, the GnRH pulses need to be timed or they can get everything off. But these pulses are going to be sensitive to environmental factors, and if you are not careful, they are going to be thrown off with fasting. Even some short term fasting, such as three days, can alter these pulses in some women.

Why does intermittent fasting affect women more than men?

This is not entirely clear yet. Many believe that it has something to do with kisspeptin, a molecule that the neurons will use to communicate with each other to get stuff down in the body. This kisspeptin is going to stimulate product of GnRH in both sexes and it can be very sensitive to ghrelin, insulin, and leptin, the hormones that will regulate and react to satiety and hunger.

What is interesting is that females often produce more of this kisspeptin than males. The more kisspeptin neurons that are in the body, the greater sensitivity there is to changes in energy balance. This could be a big reason why females are going to have more trouble with fasting.

For many women, the solution is to cut down on how long your fasting window is. Many men are able to do the Warrior diet or do alternate day fasting, but this may be a bit intense for most women, especially when you get started. You may want to consider working with either a 5:2 diet or do the 16/8 diet. These are less extreme when you first get started so your body can get used to the idea, without a big shock to the system. If you respond well to those and want to move over to alternate day fasting or another option over time, then you can consider it when you know how your body will react.

When should I consider stopping intermittent fasting?

There are times when you will want to consider stopping an intermittent fast. Even if you follow some of the advice that we give in this chapter, you may want to stop intermittent fasting if it is not working for you. Most women are going to do well with an intermittent fast if they are careful and don't fast for too long. But other women are more sensitive to the changes in their hormones, and intermittent fasting can make this worse. Some of the signs that you should consider stopping intermittent fasting include:

- You feel cold all the time.
- You can notice if your digestion is slowing down.
- You interest in romance fizzles and you don't really appreciate it at all.
- Your heart starts to feel rapid and pitter patter in a strange way.
- You see a lot of mood swings suddenly.
- You notice that your tolerance to any type of stress has decreased.
- When you get an injury, you are slow to heal, or you get a bug every time it comes around.
- When you finish with a workout, you aren't recovering as well as you should.

- You start to develop a lot of acne or dry skin.
- Your hair starts to fall out.
- You aren't able to fall asleep very well and you have trouble staying asleep.
- Your menstrual cycle becomes irregular or you find that it stops completely.

Chapter 10: The Basics of Meal Planning to Make the Fast Easier

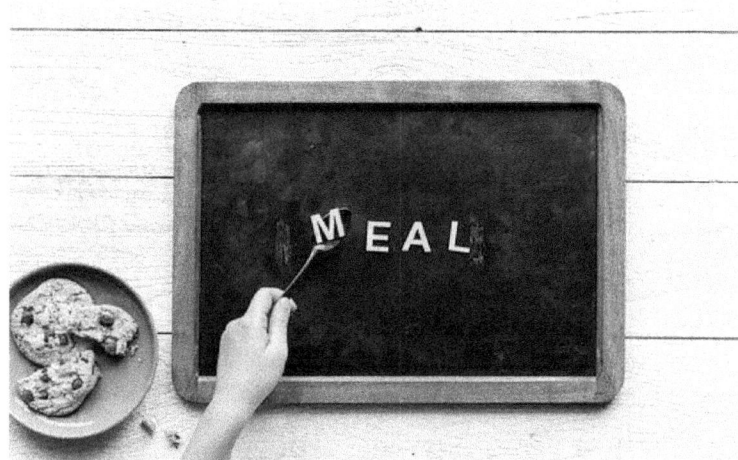

Meal planning is a way that you can organize yourself for the week when it comes to meals. Whether you make just dinners for the week or you plan out all the meals for the week and all the snacks, you are working with meal planning. Some people will plan out once a month in advance, freezing their meals and having everything ready when they need it. Others will plan out just a day in advance, although this can make it more difficult to stick with the diet plan that you are on.

Many people find that meal planning for one week at a time is easier. This helps them to make sure that they are prepared for every meal, no matter how busy they are. Fasting can be a great way to lose weight and improve your health, but when you get off the fast, you could end up binging and having trouble with what you eat if you don't have a plan.

You have to take the time to do what works the best for you. Some people want to do a week, and others like to sit down and do the whole month at a time to make things easier. Whatever method you like to use, you need to sit down and come up with the meals that work the best for you. Pick healthy meals that have a lot of nutrition and get as much work done as possible ahead of time. This can help you have a plan when you get to the fast and will ensure that you are prepared, even on your busy nights.

The benefits of meal planning

Meal planning has been growing in popularity over the past few years. People like how it can save them time and money and that it will help them to stay on a diet plan as well. There are a lot of benefits that come from adding meal planning into your life, especially when you are trying to do well with intermittent fasting. Some of the benefits that you will be able to enjoy when you start with meal planning includes:

- You will eat out less often: Many times, we go out to eat because we are too tired to make a meal at home. We could end up eating too late or taking in too many calories and throwing our intermittent fast out the door. When you have some meals ready to eat at home, this is no longer a problem that you have to worry about.

- You won't eat as many prepackaged meals. This goes along the same line as eating out. When you are in a hurry to eat at night, you may throw something in the oven or in the microwave that is not all that healthy for the body. This may make the meal fast, but it makes it very unhealthy. With some prepared meals, you can throw a few into the freezer and then have them ready when you are in a hurry.

- Your grocery store trips will be better: When you go to the grocery store, you will be able to get all the groceries that are needed for each meal. You won't get home and hope that things turn out the right way. You already know that you have the right ingredients and then you can get the meal done.

- You will be able to save a lot of money. You won't spend money on processed meals or eating out, which is going to help you save a ton of money.

- You can make sure that you eat a lot of variety in your meals. You can pick out your meals and separate out what you want each day, which ensures that you aren't stuck eating the same things all the time.

- When you get to pick out your meals ahead of time and you aren't eating out or eating a lot of prepackaged foods, you are going to be healthier. Meal planning is the perfect tool if you want to lose weight and get healthier.

- You can make sure that everyone in the family will have a say in what they get to eat. Your kids will be able to pick what they would like to eat, which could cut out some of the hassle that comes with dinner time.

- Plan for those days that are really busy: There are those days when it is almost impossible to get to the kitchen and eat at a decent time. But you can work with meal planning to cover those nights. You can put something in the slow cooker and have it there and ready on those busy nights when you just won't be able to get the meal done any other way.
- Less stress in your life: It can be stressful to come up with an idea of what to eat for supper when you are tired at the end of the day. When you decide to go with meal planning, you never have to stress out about what you will make for supper, and this can take a little bit of stress out of your day.

- Less trips heading to the grocery store: This can save you a lot of time, and even more money. You won't have to drive back and forth as much, and you run into fewer impulse buys when you do this.

Each family chooses to go with meal planning for their own personal reasons. But no matter what the reason is for you, meal planning can make life easier, can make it easier to stay on your intermittent fast, and ensures that you get a lot of healthy and delicious meals for the day.

Tips for healthy meal planning

With all the benefits of meal planning, you may be excited to get started. But you need to have a plan in place to help you get started. Some of the tips you can follow to help you get started with meal planning in your life include:

- Spend a bit of time looking for the recipes: It doesn't have to take a long time, but spending time looking for recipes can make all the difference. You can search through some of your old favorites or you can go with something new, but search the ones that you want to use, and then save them someplace safe to have during your planning day. You can set aside any day that you would like to do this but come up with enough recipes to cover either a week, two weeks, or a month, so you are ready to do all the rest of the planning that you need.

- Ask those in your home what they would enjoy eating: When you are making your meal plan, consider what some others in your home may like to eat. This can help you get more inspired and gives you more options.

- Check out the weather: The weather can make a big difference on the types of meals that you want to make for your family. If you see that the weather is going to cool down in the middle of the week, you may want to consider making some soups or working with your slow cooker. Or you may see that it is going to warm up soon and then you will choose to do some grilling. The weather can be a great way to help you get some inspiration for your meals.

- Keep a journal about your meals: It is hard to remember all the recipes that you try out and which ones you like and which ones you don't ever want to have again. Keep a meal journal, either online or writing it out, to help you remember what kinds of recipes you really liked so you can use them later on.
- Try some theme nights: One way to make picking out recipes easier is to go with a theme night. You can have a soup night, a pasta night, a slow cooker night, a Mexican night and so on. This way, you know exactly which recipes you want to go with each night of the week.

- Choose a day for shopping and make your shopping list: Pick one day out of the year when you want to go out and get all the supplies for your meal plan. And make sure that you go in with a good shopping list. This helps you to stay on track and can make the shopping trip go more smoothly.

- Check to see what the sales are: Some people like to try to save money when they are meal prepping and they will work to organize their meals around what is on sale. Check the newspaper and your favorite sales to help you figure out the meal plan that is best for you.

- Plan your leftovers: Many times, you will make a meal that will have a few leftovers. You have to figure out what your tolerance for leftovers is. sometimes you can make a big casserole and eat that for lunch for the rest of the week, and others can only do it once. Either way, try to make a bit extra of things so that you have some leftovers that you can either have again or freezer for later.

- When you get back from the store, start to prep your food: You can wash off and dry the lettuce, chop up the vegetables, and brown up the beef that you get. This way, it all gets done right away and you don't have to worry about doing it later.

- Don't overstuff your fridge too much: You may think that it is great to get the fridge stocked up as much as possible, but when you do this, some things are going to be lost behind others. By the time you get there, you are going to wonder how old that thing is and will probably need to throw it out. You can consider keeping a list nearby of all the food that is in your fridge, so you know exactly what is there and can check each thing off as you use them.

Chapter 11: Easy Ways to Keep Your Hunger at Bay During Your Fasting Window

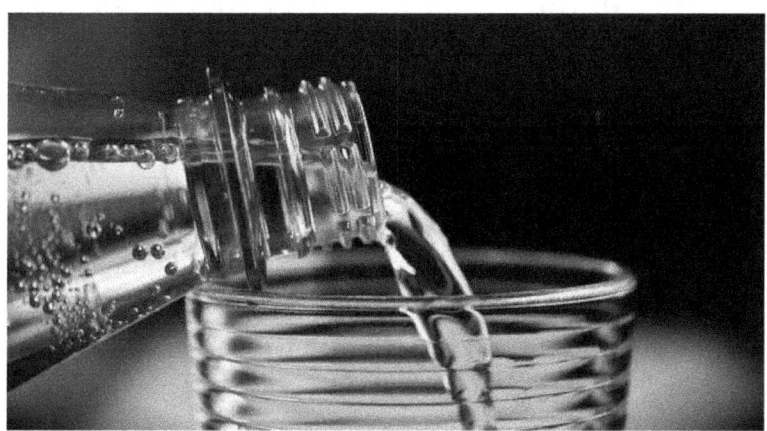

When you first get started on an intermittent fast, you are going to notice there are times when you feel hungry. It is hard to adjust the schedule of your body to get used to this way of eating and those hunger pains can be hard to ignore.There are a few things that you can do to help keep those hunger pains away, so you can get the full benefits of being on an intermittent fast without feeling miserable the whole time.

Drink more water and keep yourself hydrated

The first thing that you should try to do is drink more water. Often, those pains that we associate with being hungry are just pains to be thirsty and we just need to drink more water in our diet. You should aim for between eight to ten glasses a day, but if you are really active, you may need to add in some more glasses to help you stay hydrated. Learn how to listen to your body so you get enough water to help you out.

Regular water can be really nice and it works for a lot of people. But if you are drinking plenty of water and you see that you are still hungry, you may want to try carbonated water. Many people are going to find that the bubbles in this kind of water can make all the difference and can help fill you up. Keep a few of these around the house for when you are really hungry and you need to make it a little bit longer before eating.

Slow down your eating

It takes the body some time to digest the food that you are taking in. if you gobble up all of the meals that you eat while on an intermittent fast, you are going to miss out on feeling full and eating fewer calories. Then, you may still feel hungry, even when it is time to fast and you just ate. Slowing down how fast you decide to eat can make a big difference in how hungry you feel during the day and how long you will be able to maintain your fast.

It takes the brain about twenty minutes to realize it is full. But if you are scarfing down your food as fast as you can, you could eat a ton of calories in that twenty minutes and really make yourself uncomfortable. But if you learn to take things slower, you will realize when you are full and can learn how to listen to your body, then you may start to see that those hunger pains are more about being bored, or thirsty, or something else rather than being hungry.

Eat plenty of fiber and protein in your meals

The right amount of certain nutrients can make a big difference in how hungry you are going to feel. When the body is missing out on these important nutrients, it becomes really hard to avoid those hunger cues, and you may not be able to stay on your intermittent fast very well.

The first nutrient that you need to make sure you get plenty of in this fast is fiber. Fiber is great for filling up the stomach, so you can take in fewer calories while still feeling like you ate a full meal. In addition, this fiber is able to clean out the digestive tract, so you are able to take on a detox at the same time.

Another important nutrient that you can consider is taking in plenty of protein. Many diet plans that you go with will talk about getting some protein into your diet. This nutrient is able to help you get more your hormones in order and most foods that are high in protein are very filling as well. Try to add a bit of protein into your meals and see what a difference it can do with your hunger pains.

Get enough sleep at night

You need to make sure that you get enough sleep during the night. The amount of sleep that you choose to get each night is going to direction affect how hungry you feel while you are fasting. When you don't get enough sleep during the night, the hormones in your body will get all messed up. Not only will you get tired, but the body will convince you that you are starving, even if you have gotten enough calories.

Even if you were able to make it until the end of your fasting window, you are going to have a hard day when your eating window opens up. You may find that you have a lot of cravings and it is really hard to stop eating once you have started. your day, and your diet plan, are going to be ruined if you don't get enough sleep into your day.

It is best to try and sleep enough at night. This can help you to feel better, feel more fit, and can help you stay away from those cravings that could ruin your intermittent fast. Getting eight to nine hours at night is the best, but if your schedule doesn't allow for this, you may want to consider finding room to take a small nap during the day to get enough sleep.

Have a little bit of soup before one of your meals

If you are worried about keeping yourself full and healthy, you may want to consider adding in a little bit of soup with your meals. Some soup can be really filling and will make sure that you stay within your calorie allotment without having to feel hungry all the time. Soup can work as a nice snack before your meal or have it right at the end of your eating window so you stay fuller for longer. Try to pick out soups that have a lot of nutrients, such as vegetable and beef soup, so you can really make your body happy before you go into a fast.

Light a candle that smells like vanilla

Have you ever heard of something that is known as Christmas Dinner Syndrome? This is when the person who has been cooking the meal all day isn't going to eat as much as the other guests. This is usually because they spent all their day smelling the dinner. The theory here is that the sweet scents can reduce sugar cravings and will keep hunger at bay. Vanilla is often a good scent to go with to help you keep hunger away. You can choose to light it before your fast is over, or you can just sniff the candle and see if that can help.

Think about the color of your plate

As strange as it may sound, you will find that the color of your plate can make a big difference in how much food that you eat. If you go with a warm color like orange or red, you are more likely to eat more. But if you go with a cool color, especially blue, you will eat less. It doesn't seem to matter what size the plate is. There is something in the brain that reacts differently to the warm colors versus the cool colors. So, take a look at your dishes and consider updating to something in a cooler color, at least for supper, to help turn off the appetite before you go into your fast.

Take a picture of your meal

You can just do it for your own personal use or you can Instagram it and share it with friends and family. This may seem a little silly or a little self-centered, you may be able to use it as a tool to eat healthier on your intermittent fast. It not only concentrates the mind on eating healthier foods, but less of it, which can help with weight loss overall. And it seems that this kind of photograph is going to deter any binges that you may feel like going on.

Call up a friend

When you are feeling hungry, consider calling up a friend and talking with them for a little bit. This can help provide you with a good distraction during the day and can keep you away from food for a bit longer. In addition, research shows that when you hear a kind or familiar voice, it can stimulate your brain to release oxytocin, a stress fighting, mood boosting, love hormone. When you feel less stress, this can help to increase your satiety hormone, leptin. So, keep a list of close friends and family members nearby so you can call them up when the hunger pangs start to get strong.

Add some greens to your water

One thing that you can try is not only drink water, but also considering adding in a teaspoon or so of some super greens to your water. Not only can this help to boost how many nutrients you are taking in, including wheat grass, barley, chlorella, and spirulina, but they have fiber that can help you feel fuller for longer. Add in that they also contain a lot of nutrients that help give you energy, and it is no wonder that a lot of people like to have some greens with their water during the day.

If you don't like having some of those super greens during the day, you can consider having some tea. Adding two to three cups of green tea can help you to keep hunger away and can make it easier to lose weight than ever before. The catechins that are inside green tea are also perfect for balancing out your levels of blood sugars. Add onto that how green tea can help to lower your triglycerides and cholesterol so it is extra good for you. You can have a little non-caloric green tea during your fast when you feel hungry.

Do your exercise routine during your fasting window, a few hours before you can eat

While it may sound counterintuitive, you will find that a little bit of exercise can make the difference in how hungry you feel. Getting in some moderate exercise can be enough to turn those hunger cues down so you can make it through the rest of your fasting window. You don't want to overdo this, or you will get really hungry and will overindulge when the fasting window happens. But doing about thirty minutes of a workout can make a big difference on your appetite and can make those hunger pains go away.

A good time to do your workout is when you notice that your body is getting hungry. If you are going the 16/8 diet plan, you may start to feel hungry an hour or so after your regular breakfast. But you may still have a few hours before you are able to consume anything when the eating window opens up. Instead of feeling miserable or cheating and eating something during your fasting window, you can consider doing a workout.

When you feel hungry, the last thing you want to do is try to do a workout. But you may find that going on a walk or lifting a few weights not only helps to improve your health and makes it easier to lose weight, but it can also help make the hunger go away. Just spend half an hour or so and you will see a big difference in your levels of hunger and it will be easier to make it through the rest of the fast.

One of the hardest things that you will have to deal with when you get started with intermittent fasting is those hunger pains as the body adapts to this new eating cycle. Over time, you will get used to it and may only feel those hunger pains on occasion. Until that happens, go ahead and try out some of these tips to make things easier.

Chapter 12: Setting Up a Support Group to Keep You on Track

When you go on an intermittent fast, or any kind of diet or eating plan, you may find that you feel lonely when you first start. You may feel like there is no one else who is dieting at that time and that you are the only one out there that is dealing with this. You may be invited to parties, have events at work, or have other things that go on in your life that can make it difficult to stick to the diet. And every day life can make it hard to stick with an intermittent fast, no matter how hard you try.

If you try to do an intermittent fast on your own, it is more likely that you are going to fail with it. This is because it is hard to hold yourself accountable all the time. If no one is checking in on you, you may feel lonely, you may feel that it is not such a big deal to cheat on occasion, and before you know it, you have gone off the diet and missed out on all the great benefits that come with this type of eating plan.

A better option to go with is to find some kind of support group that you can work with. Support groups can be there in all sorts of situations. You may have them there to ask advice from, to share success and failures with, and to hold you accountable when things get a little bit tough. Each person on an intermittent fast, or any other diet plan, should consider finding a good support group that can help them out.

There are many different types of support groups that you can choose to join. You can go with a close friend or family member who is also looking to improve their health. This is often the best type of support group that you can choose because they are the closest to you and want you to succeed. You can go to the gym together, talk to each other when someone is feeling hungry and like giving up with their fasting time, and someone to hold you accountable during every step of the process. You could get a whole group of your family and friends together to help you stick with your intermittent fast and everyone can improve their health in the process.

If you don't have any friends or family who are willing to work with you on intermittent fasting in your friends and family group, look around your local town and see what options there are. You may run into trouble finding people who are specifically doing an intermittent fast, but you may be able to join a group where people are dieting in general. They can still provide you with advice and help to keep you on track with your fasting schedule.

For most people, finding a support group online is going to be the way that they get this done. This allows them to reach people from all over the place, offering more support and opportunity to ask more questions. You can share ideas on recipes, talk to people who have been in intermittent fasting for a long time and those who have just began, and so much more. This is a place to be open with yourself and make sure that you are getting the most out of your fast. Make sure to look around and find the one that is perfect for your needs.

How can a social support system help you lose weight?

It won't take long for you to find that it is easier to stick with a weight loss plan and stay on your intermittent fast when you have support. This support can come in many forms and will help you when you need tips on dieting, exercise, and staying accountable for your actions. There are a lot of different places where you are going to be able to find this support, but some of the best options will include:

Informal commercial programs

These kinds of programs are going to rely on support from a group, discussions about diet and exercise, and even some assignments, such as keeping a food diary. These are great options for a lot of different people because it holds them accountable and lets them have a chance to get out and be social with other people along the way.

In one study, researchers looked to see how the Weight Watchers program, with regular meetings and social support, worked against the self-help approach. The self-help approach consists of two small sessions with a dietician and some printed materials that you can use to help keep yourself on track. In this study, researchers found that those who were in Weight Watchers were able to lose over three times the pounds compared to those in the self-help group just in the first year.

On average, those who were in the Weight Watchers group would like an average of ten pounds compared to the three pounds that those in the self-help group. By the end of the second year, both groups had regained some weight. The self-help group went back to their starting weight, but most of the participants in Weight Watchers were able to keep off at least six pounds, so they were still less than when they started.

This shows that Weight Watchers and other similar social group programs may be a great option for you when you are trying to lose weight. They help you get some support from others who are in the same kind of situation, and you get held accountable for your actions with the weekly meetings. For many people, this is a great way to stay healthy and see better results.

Clinic based groups

Another option that you may want to consider is to do a clinic-based group for intermittent fasting or for weight loss. Many of these are going to be based on groups and will occur at a medical center or at a local university depending on where you live.

These groups are going to be run by a variety of professionals, including those who work with weight loss, nutritionists, and psychologists. These programs are going to last for a set number of weeks, so you know exactly what you are getting into with the program. Thanks to the individualized attention that you can get with these courses, these groups can often lead to more weight loss compared to the commercial programs. There has yet to be research or studies done on which one is better, but many people believe that the professional help and personalized approach can make these a better option if you need to lose weight quickly and efficiently.

A Trevose Behavior Modification Program

This kind of program came out in 1970 and was started by a formerly obese person and an obesity researcher. This is a very rigorous type of program that will require you to go to weekly group sessions if you want to do well. You will also need to meet some weight loss goals that you and a nutritionist agreed on together or you might be kicked out of the group.

One benefit of this group is that because it is run by volunteers, it is a free program and even though it is pretty hard core compared to the others, it does seem to work. In one study, participants were able to lose at least 19 percent of their body weight in just two years, which is more than the other two options were able to do. And these participants were able to keep that weight off for the long term.

After five years, the participants that went on this program were still about 17 percent from their initial weight, which is much better than other programs. However, this kind of approach can sometimes be too much for many participants. In one study to see how effective this method was, just under half of those who originally started were still doing the program after two years.

Social support

While a lot of these programs can be successful, there is still a problem with how people will be able to keep that weight off when they are done with group treatment. Studies show that enlisting friends and family with this effort may help. In one study, those who went into a weight loss program with friends would do a better job keeping that weight off.

In addition to being able to team up with their friends, these enrollees were given social support along with the regular treatment that comes with those programs. Two-thirds of those who enrolled with a friend were able to keep that weight off up to six months after the meetings stopped. Those who didn't attend with a friend were not able to do the same thing, with only a quarter of those participants being successful.

As you can see, there are many different methods that you can use in order to help you gain the support that you need to stick with an intermittent fast and see results. Pick out the one that works the best for you and see how great an intermittent fast can be!

Chapter 13: The Other Side of Intermittent Fasting – The Side Effects and Who Shouldn't Go on an Intermittent Fast

While intermittent fasting is a great type of eating plan to go on, there are some times when you may have to deal with a few side effects. These side effects are usually minor, and they won't last very long. If you are able to get through about a week or two on an intermittent fast, you will be able to leave these side effects behind and feel better. It is still a good idea to know about these side effects and what they can mean for you. Some of the most common side effects that come with an intermittent fast include:

Hunger

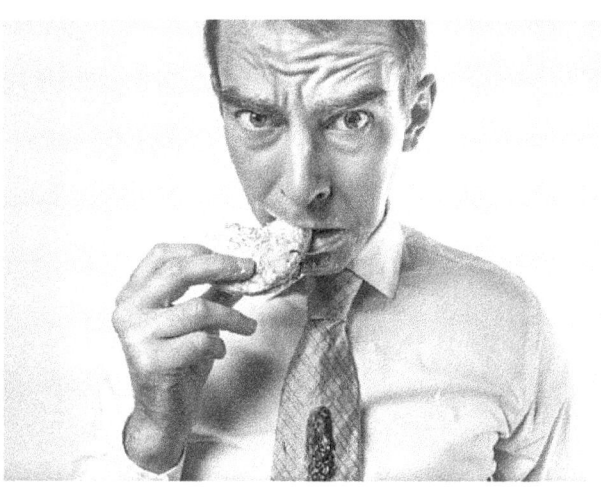

When your body is used to being able to eat five or six times a day, it starts to expect food at certain times. The ghrelin hormone is the one that is in charge of making us feel hungry. It is going to peak best at breakfast, lunch, and dinner, and it is regulated, at least in part, by the food that we take in. when you first start with fasting, your ghrelin levels will still peak, and you will still feel hungry during meal times. Often days three to five will feel the worst. But if you can stick with this schedule, those peaks are going to fall away, and you may even have days when the eating window is coming to an end and you aren't even feeling hungry at all.

The best thing that you can do to combat hunger and make yourself feel better as you get through your fasting window is to drink a lot of water. This helps you to feel more alert, can keep the belly full, and can help fulfil the need to put something in your mouth when you feel hungry.

You may also find that drinking tea or black coffee can be a great way to curb hunger. Keep busy, avoidworkouts that are too strenuous, and get enough sleep.

When you are in your eating window, making sure that you eat enough and get plenty of good protein, healthy fats, and carbs can make a difference in how hungry you are going to be the next day.

Cravings

When you are told that you aren't allowed to do something, chances are that the thing you will want to do the most is that one thing. Doesn't matter what that thing is, we are set up that way. When you are on an intermittent fast, there are times when you will go an extra-long time without getting to eat anything. Many people find that because of this, they are only able to think about eating and how much they miss eating.

This is when those cravings are going to start kicking in. During your fasting window, you are more likely to want refined carbs and sweets, mostly because the body is missing out on that easy source of energy and it wants to get that glucose hit right away.

To make this part easier, you need to find ways to distract yourself. Do what you can to not think about food. You can go and do some exercise, you can visit with friends and family, you can clean the house, or even get work done. Then, when it is time to get back into your eating window, make sure that you slightly indulge those cravings to get them to go away. You don't want to let them take over too much, but a little bit won't harm anything and can make you feel better after a fast.

Headaches

As your body starts to get used to eating in this new manner, there are times when you may get a dull headache that kind of comes and goes. One reason for this could be from dehydration as you may forget to drink enough when you aren't eating enough. Make sure that you keep a bottle of water full and right next to you the whole time. That way, you have a constant reminder that you need another drink before it's too late.

In addition to dehydration, it is possible that these headaches are going to be caused when your levels of blood sugars decrease. Or it could be from some of the stress hormones that the brain will release when you go on a fast. The good news is that your body is going to get used to this new way of eating, you just need to give it some time. You need to keep yourself as stress-free as possible during this time, and maybe find a way to relax and take some good pain relievers to help you while the body adjusts.

Low energy

During the first few days on an intermittent fast, remember that you are going to be a little bit low on energy. This can make staying on an intermittent fast a bit harder, but as your body adjusts, you will be able to feel that your levels of energy do go up, you just have to give it time.

The issue here is that the body is used to getting a constant source of fuel from you when you choose to eat all day long. Once you take this away, the body is going to feel a bit sluggish as it tries to figure out where to get that fuel and as it has to start doing more of the work on its own.

The best thing that you can do here is work to keep your day as relaxing as possible. Exert as little energy as possible. Many people will choose to avoid their workouts during the first few weeks to help keep them relaxed and get the body adjusted. If you do decide to workout, go with workouts like yoga or light walking. You can also consider some extra sleep and taking some naps to make this easier.

Irritability

As you get used to not eating for longer periods of time, you are going to feel hungry. And when you feel hungry and angry, it can be really hard to deal with. During at least the first few days of this diet plan, expect that you are going to feel a little bit cranky when you have a blood sugar drop. And some of the other side effects that come with intermittent fasting can make things hard as well. Low energy, hunger, lots of cravings, heartburn and more can all make you a little bit angry and hard to be around.

The best thing to do during the first week or so on an intermittent fast is to figure out how you can avoid situations and people that already annoy you, because the situation is just going to be worse for a few days. Try to focus on doing something every day that helps make you happy, so you are better able to deal with this irritability.

Constipation, bloating, and heartburn

When you are eating and digesting food, the stomach is going to produce some acid to help with this. The body gets used to your normal periods of eating, which is often all the time on a traditional American diet. This means that it is constantly producing acid to help you digest your food. But when you stop eating all the time and start doing periods of fasting, it may take the body some time to adjust and stop making so much acid.

This could result in issues like heartburn, bloating and constipation. Out of these, heartburn is one that isn't as common as the others, but it may be something that you have to consider when you first get started. it could range from some mild discomfort to burping all day or even full on pain. The best thing to do for this is take some antacids and realize that time is going to help cure this issue.

To avoid heart burn and constipation, make sure that you drink a lot of water, prop yourself up when you go to sleep for the night, and try to avoid any foods that will make the heartburn worse, such as greasy and spicy foods. If you are on the intermittent fast for some time and it doesn't feel like the heartburn or constipation are going away, you may want to go and discuss this issue with your doctor.

Feeling cold

Some people who go on an intermittent fast will notice that they feel colder when they first start. Cold fingers and toes can be pretty common when you are fasting, but there is a good reason for this. When you are fasting, the blood flow in the body is going to start heading to the fat stores. This is known as adipose tissue blood flow. And while it results in some colder fingers and toes for a bit, it is actually going to help the body move fat over to your muscles so that it can be used up as fuel.

This may make you a little bit chilly and uncomfortable when you first get started, but it is really doing a great thing. Your body is working to move the fat from you and turn it into fuel that can burn quickly. It may make you a bit more sensitive to the cold, but it helps give you the trim and lean look that you want. You can combat some of this coldness simply by sipping hot tea, wearing some extra layers, avoiding the cold for longer periods of time, and taking warm showers to help.

Overeating

Another issue that you may face is that you may overeat when you are done with your fasting window. People tend to overeat after they have been on a fast because they are really hungry and are trying to make up for the lost calories. There are a few reasons why you may overeat when you are on your intermittent fast journey. Often it is because people believe that when they are fasting, the calories aren't going to matter, even though they do. Or people may overeat because they are so excited to finally be able to eat that they tend to overdo it when it's time to eat.

Planning out your meals ahead of time can be one of the best things that you can do. This helps you to keep your portions in check and will ensure that you aren't taking in more calories than you should after finishing up your fast.

Many people find that they are going to feel almost famished when they get to their eating window. They will then choose to eat really fast, faster than they normally would. This can really end up with a lot more calories in the diet than normal and can make it hard to get the good benefits of an intermittent fast. When you get done with your fasting window and enter the eating window, you must be mindful about that first meal. Eat slowly, pick meals that are high in nutrients, and learn how to really listen to your body so you stop eating when you are full.

Bathroom trips

This issue usually isn't that big of a deal. But since you will probably drink a lot of extra water to make sure that you are hydrated and that you are filled up, you may have to run and make more bathroom trips than before. There isn't really a way to get around this because you still want to make sure that you take in plenty of water when you are on an intermittent fast. Over time, you will get used to this and it won't be that big of a deal.

There are times when you will run into trouble with an intermittent fast. There are some side effects that can make it a bit harder to follow this kind of diet plan, and many people worry about how the first few weeks will be. But while there are some side effects that you need to worry about, they aren't as bad as some other options, and after a week or two, they will usually fade away. If you can just stick with the eating plan for a little bit, you are going to get the great results without all the bad side effects.

Chapter 14: Common Myths About Intermittent Fasting

With the rise in popularity with intermittent fasting, there have been a few myths popping up all over the place. People worry about skipping breakfast and how it will affect their metabolism. They worry that intermittent fasting will be too hard for them to follow. Some even worry that intermittent fasting is going to be bad for their health and will make them lose muscle tone if they do it more than a few days.

But many of these topics, and more, are simply myths about our health. And listening to them can make us miss out on some of the great benefits that come with an intermittent fast. Let's take a look at some of the most common myths that come with intermittent fasting and why we need to be careful about what we believe.

Skipping breakfast can make you fat

It is a long-held belief that eating breakfast is the most important meal of the day. it is so prevalent that many people believe that if they skip breakfast, they are going to have cravings, excessive hunger, and weight gain. While there are some observational studies that show how skipping breakfast and being overweight can be linked, this is often explained by the fact that the breakfast skipper is often not very health conscious to start with.

There was one study done in 2014 that compared skipping breakfast versus eating breakfast in 283 adults who were either overweight or obese. After the 16 weeks of the study, there wasn't a difference in weight with the two groups. This shows that it doesn't make a difference in weight loss whether you choose to eat breakfast or not.

There are some studies that do show that eating breakfast for some individuals may be a good thing. Teenagers who ate breakfast tended to do better when they were at school. And some people who lose weight in the long term, showing that they tend to eat breakfast to lose the weight. This can vary depending on the individual person. If you need breakfast to keep your eating in check, you can choose to change your eating window to include breakfast and quit eating earlier in the evening. This is a simple change that can make intermittent fasting work for you.

Eating frequent meals can help boost up your metabolism

Many people follow the idea that eating many small meals is what is needed to keep that metabolism moving fast. They believe that when you eat more meals, it is going to increase your metabolic rate so that the calories burnt by the body are more overall.

It is true that when the body is digesting and assimilating nutrients in your meal, it is going to use up some energy. This is called the thermic effect of food. This ends you being about twenty to thirty percent of your calories for protein, five to ten percent for carbs, and then up to three percent for fat calories.

For most meals you eat, this thermic effect is going to be about ten percent of calories that you take in. The important thing to remember here is that the total calories consumed is what matters, not the number of meals you eat them in. eating six five hundred calorie meals is going to have the same effect on the body as eating three 1000 calorie meals. You will get the same thermic effect.

This works the other way around as well. You can decrease your meals and still get the same thermic effect of food, as long as you eat the same, or similar, numbers of calories. Increasing or decreasing how often you eat meals will have no effect on how many calories you burn altogether.

Small and frequent meals are necessary to lose weight

This is another recent fad that has come around in the dieting world, but one that doesn't really hold much basis. Frequent meals have not been shown to increase your metabolism and they aren't really that affective at reducing hunger in the body. In fact, most studies find that the amount of meals that you consume during the day will not affect how much weight you can lose.

In one study that followed 16 obese women and men, there wasn't any difference in weight, appetite, and fat loss when comparing how things went when they ate either three or six meals each day. So, you may be eating all those meals without getting any benefits.

The brain needs to always have a supply of glucose to function

This myth relies on the idea that the brain needs to have carbs and glucose all the time, or it will stop working. This idea only works if you believe that the brain is only able to use blood sugar for fuel. This is just not true. First, the body can work with the glycogen that is stored in the body as body fat to help fuel the bran. Second, the brain can use ketones, or the dietary fats that you consume or that are in the body, as fuel as well.

It just doesn't make sense from an evolutionary perspective that we wouldn't be able to make it without that constant source of carbs to help us out. While some people have trouble with hypoglycemia if they don't eat for a while, most people will be just fine on a fast.

Fasting will put the body into starvation mode

One common myth that people make against intermittent fasting, and fasting in general, is that it will put the body into starvation mode. This claim says that when you don't eat, you are making the body think that it is starving. When the body thinks that you are starving, it will shut down, or at least slow down, the metabolism and make it hard to burn any fat.

While it is true that losing weight over the long-term can reduce how many calories that you burn each day, this is something that can happen with any type of weight loss program you go on. It is a natural process that the body goes through called adaptive thermo genesis. And there are even some studies that show how a short-term fast can increase your metabolic rate.

Some studies show how fasting for a period that is no more than 48 hours can actually help to boost your metabolism by 3.6 to 14 percent. However, if you fast for a longer period than this, it could put your body into that "starvation mode" and your metabolism will slow down. So, the amount of time that you fast can make a difference. Luckily, all the options for intermittent fasting ask you to only go for 24 hours, at most, so you can increase the metabolism without having to worry about cutting as many calories.

Intermittent fasting can make me lose muscle

It is a common misconception that intermittent fasting is going to make you lose muscle. Those who believe this one think that the body is going to automatically resort to using muscle to fuel it when you go for a few hours without eating. This can happen with any type of dieting plan and doesn't happen anymore with intermittent fasting than the others. There are even some studies that show how intermittent fasting can be better for you if you want to maintain your muscle mass.

In one particular review study, restricting calorie consumption intermittently caused a similar amount of weight loss as doing a calorie restriction diet, but the muscle mass reduction wasn't as severe.

In another study, the participants would eat the same number of calories that they usually did for two meals. But then in the evening they were supposed to eat one huge meal. These people lost body fat and helped create a modest increase in their muscle mass. They also had a lot of other beneficial health markers.

Another proof that intermittent fasting isn't going to make you lose your body muscle mass? Many bodybuilders like to use intermittent fasting. They find that this is an easy and effective method to help them to maintain high amounts of muscle with a low body fat percentage.

Intermittent fasting can be bad for your health

There are some people who refuse to go on an intermittent fast because they think this kind of fasting is harmful to their health. There are many studies out there that show how intermittent fasting, and intermittent calorie restriction, can have some impressive benefits to your health. For example, intermittent fasting has the power to change how the genes related to longevity will express themselves.

Doing a good intermittent fast can also help reduce factors that can cause heart disease, reduces inflammation, and can improve your insulin sensitivity. Some use it to help boost their brains power by boosting the hormone known as BDNF, or brain-derived neurotrophic factor. This hormone may be the link to help fight off depression and other brain problems.

So, while some people worry that intermittent fasting is going to ruin their health and make them feel miserable, the studies behind this are just not there. Intermittent fasting, in any form that you choose, can make a positive difference in your health and can help you get in the best shape of your life.

Intermittent fasting will make you overeat

There are some who claim that intermittent fasting isn't going to cause weight loss because when you reach your eating window, you will naturally overeat. While it is true that many people tend to overeat a little bit more after a fast to help compensate for that time without food. However, this isn't a complete compensation. One study showed how people who fasted for a whole day still only ended up with 500 extra calories on the following day.

So, if you went all day without eating during your first and you normally eat 2000 calories a day, even with the extra 500 calories on that non-fasting day, you averaged 1250 for the two days. That is still enough of a calorie cut to help you lose weight.

Being on an intermittent fast means that you are reducing your overall food intake while still boosting your metabolism. It can also reduce your insulin levels, boosts the human growth hormone, and can increase norepinephrine, which can make it easier for you to lose weight.

In fact, intermittent fasting can really help you lose a lot of weight faster than any other diet plan. According to a review study that was done in 2014, fasting over a period of 3 to 24 weeks could cause the participant to lose three to eight percent in body weight. They also saw a reduction between 4 to 7 percent in their belly fat, which alone can help reduce a whole host of health conditions.

Intermittent fasting is not going to make you overeat overall. In fact, it can help to reduce the amount of food that you take in and reduce how many calories you consume. After a fast, you may overcompensate for the first meal or two, but this overcompensation is not going to be enough to throw your whole day of fasting out the window.

Conclusion

Thank you for making it through to the end of *Intermittent Fasting for Beginners*, let's hope it was informative and able to provide you with all the tools you need to achieve your goals whatever they may be.

The next step is to set up your plan to help you get started with intermittent fasting. There are so many choices when you decide that intermittent fasting is the right choice for you. So, the first step is to pick out the type of intermittent fast that you want to go on, and then move on from there to pick out an exercise program that you like and to stick with a meal plan that will help you get the right nutrition, even when you are fasting.

This guidebook took some time to look through the different parts of intermittent fasting so you are able to make an informed decision about whether this is the right option for you or not. We looked at what intermittent fasting is all about, why it is such a good option to go with to improve your health, how to set up a meal plan and an exercise program that can help enhance your results, and how to get the most out of this eating plan.

While there are a lot of different diet programs out there, none can compete with the great benefits you can get from an intermittent fast. Check out this guidebook to get all the information that you need to get started with this incredible fasting program!

Finally, if you found this book useful in anyway, a review on Amazon is always appreciated!

The Ketogenic Diet for Beginners
The Complete Guide to the Keto Diet Offering Clarity to Reset and Heal your Body

© Copyright 2018 by _____ - All rights reserved.

The following eBook is reproduced below with the goal of providing information that is as accurate and reliable as possible. Regardless, purchasing this eBook can be seen as consent to the fact that both the publisher and the author of this book are in no way experts on the topics discussed within and that any recommendations or suggestions that are made herein are for entertainment purposes only. Professionals should be consulted as needed prior to undertaking any of the action endorsed herein.

This declaration is deemed fair and valid by both the American Bar Association and the Committee of Publishers Association and is legally binding throughout the United States.

Furthermore, the transmission, duplication, or reproduction of any of the following work including specific information will be considered an illegal act irrespective of if it is done electronically or in print. This extends to creating a secondary or tertiary copy of the work or a recorded copy and is only allowed withexpress written consent from the Publisher. All additional right reserved.

The information in the following pages is broadly considered to be a truthful and accurate account of facts and as such any inattention, use or misuse of the information in question by the reader will render any resulting actions solely under their purview. There are no scenarios in which the publisher or the original author of this work can be in any fashion deemed liable for any hardship or damages that may befall them after undertaking information described herein.

Additionally, the information in the following pages is intended only for informational purposes and should thus be thought of as universal. As befitting its nature, it is presented without assurance regarding its prolonged validity or interim quality. Trademarks that are mentioned are done without written consent and can in no way be considered an endorsement from the trademark holder.

Introduction

The easiest way to explain what the Ketogenic diet is- it is a high-fat, low-carbohydrate, and medium-protein diet. When the diet was started, it was a treatment for refractory epilepsy in children. When followed, it causes the body to burn fat for energy instead of carbs.

The majority of carbohydrates people eat are changed to glucose in the body, which is transported around and helps fuel the body and the brain. However, if the body is not given enough carbohydrates, the liver will start to change fat within the body into fatty acids and ketone bodies. These ketones will then move to the brain to replace glucose. The higher level of ketones in the body is what is helping to reduce the chances of epileptic seizures in children.

Almost half of the kids that were placed on this diet ended up seeing a reduction of seizures and these effects continue even after they returned to their normal diet. With a classic keto diet, you consume about a four to one ratio by weight of combined carbohydrates and protein to fat. This is achieved by removing high-carbohydrate foods such as fruits, sugar, starchy veggies, grains, bread, and pasta. People will also increase their consumption of nuts, butter, and cream that is high in fat.

Most fats that are found in foods are LCTs or long-chain triglycerides. However, MCTs or medium-chain triglycerides are consumed more in a keto diet. Most people who follow a keto diet will consume a lot of coconut oil because it has higher levels of MCTs, or they will use MCT oil and add it to their morning cup of coffee.

Everyone's body and needs are going to be slightly different, but your macros will typically look something like this. 60 to 75 percent of your calories should come from fat, 15 to 30 percent of your calories should come from protein, and 5 to 10 percent of your calories should come from carbs.

After a person has been on a keto diet for a few days, the body will enter what is called ketosis, which we will talk about more in detail later. This is where your body will begin to use up all of your stored fat and the fat you eat for energy.

While this may have been originally used to help people who suffered from epilepsy, people began to see how useful it was to drop a few extra pounds. See, when you eat a lot of carbs, the body retains a lot of fluid so that it is able to store those carbs to use as energy. When a lot of carbs aren't consumed, you end up losing all of those stored fluids.

The biggest reason why people choose to start a diet is to get rid of their stored fats. Keto diet literally targets those areas. While in the beginning, it may seem like it would be hard to stick to because you will have to cut out a lot of different foods, there are many different creative ways to make sure that you won't miss out on some tasty meals. And if you do end up sticking with the diet, you will see that your waistline will start shrinking.

While we're on the subject of foods, there are some products out there that are aimed towards ketogenic dieters. FATBAR is a common one. They create snack bars that contain 200 calories, 16 grams of fat, and four grams of net carbs.

For people who love their morning cup of Joe and may have become used to having a vanilla latte every morning, you can switch it to a bulletproof coffee. This is a regular black coffee with a bit of added butter and MCT oil. It gives you the perfect jump of energy to get your day started.

Before we dive into the specifics of the keto diet, let's look at some differences you may be wondering about.

Keto vs. Atkins

These are the two most popular diets that reduce your carb intake drastically, but let's look at how they compare to each other in terms of results, difficulty, and safety.

The Atkins diet and the keto diet would be neck and neck in a race for the most popular low-carb diets. Both don't just cut back on the bad-for-you carbs such as cookies, donuts, and cupcakes, but they also cut out some veggies and the majority of fruits. They limit carbs enough to make you enter ketosis, which makes the body burn fat for fuel after your glucose stores have been depleted. Ketosis plays a big role in both of these diets, and it also affects how easy it is to stick with them.

Let's quickly go through the Atkins diet. It was introduced in 1972 by Robert Atkins, a cardiologist. The original form of it, which is now called Atkins 20, was made up of four phases. The first phase had the most restrictive rules.

Fats and proteins in Atkins are fair game, but carbs are extremely restrictive to between 20 and 25 grams of net carbs, which are the total carbohydrates minus the dietary fiber. All of these carbs should come from cheese, veggies, seeds, and nuts. This phase lasts until you are about 15 pounds away from your goal weight.

Phase two will bring your carb amount to 25 to 50 grams and you can add in foods like yogurt, cottage cheese, and blueberries. This will last until you are ten pounds away from your goal weight.

In phase three, you will increase your carbs to between 50 and 80 grams of net carbs while you are trying to find the best balance. This means, how many carbs are you able to eat before your weight loss stalls. This part should be done slowly and with a bit of trial and error to figure out how many carbs you can consume with gaining weight.

After you have found that number and managed to maintain it for a month, you will hit phase four. This is lifetime maintenance. This part focuses on keeping up with the habits that you developed during the third phase. You can have up to 100 grams of net carbs per day as long as you don't start gaining weight.

There are a lot of different moving parts when it comes to the Atkins diet. With the keto diet, you have only one way to eat for the complete diet. You will lower your carb intake to around five percent of your daily calorie intake. As a result, you enter ketosis and many people will monitor this by using urine strips or blood tests.

A lot of people still only recommend the keto diet for children with epilepsy because getting rid of complete food groups can drastically change the way you eat, which poses some risk. Some evidence suggests that it can help adults that have epilepsy as well, but there needs to be more research.

If not followed safely and properly, the keto diet can cause an increased risk of kidney stones and possible heart disease, as well as deficiencies in essential minerals and vitamins. In addition to that, until your body has adapted, the buildup of ketones can cause bad breath, mental fatigue, headaches, and nausea.

You will most likely lose weight on both of these diets. In the beginning, it will mainly be water weight. There is a chance with both that the water weight will be regained once you start eating normally again. Studies have found that people who followed the Atkins diet lost 4.6 to 10.3 pounds, though they regained some of that by the end of their second year.

Keto and Atkins don't make you count calories. The important thing is to make sure that you stay under your number of net carbs. Keto does need you to make sure you are hitting the right percentage of calories coming from protein and fat as well.

It depends on each individual person as to which diet is the easiest to follow. It all depends on your habits before you begin the diet. Neither of them is easy.

The main difference between these diets is the amount of protein you can consume. Atkins doesn't put a cap on your protein consumption, but keto does. The other difference is having your body in ketosis during the entire diet. Only the keto diet requires you to stay in ketosis. The Atkins diet slowly lets you reintroduce carbs.

This means that the Atkins diet may be a bit more sustainable in the long run since it is not as restrictive.

Keto vs. Paleo

Paleo is another popular diet people talk about a lot. Let's look at how these two diets compare.

The paleo diet is often called "the caveman diet" and is based on the principles of consuming foods that are available for early humans. One of the theories of the paleo diet is that our modern food systems, processing, and production techniques are harming our health. If you change your eating style to the Paleolithic hunter-gatherer, you will be able to support your own natural biological function and improve your health and digestion. Paleo gets rid of the dairy, processed sugar, legumes, and grains.

The majority of foods that paleo dieters eat are:

- Minimally processed sweetener like raw stevia, coconut sugar, maple syrup, and raw honey.
- Select fats and oils like butter/ghee, tallow, lard, avocado oil, olive oil, and coconut oil.
- Vegetables, except for corn.
- Fruits
- Seeds and nuts
- Eggs
- Fish and meat

For the majority of people who follow paleo, it has less to do with the diet and more for healthier lifestyle practices, the impact on the environment, and total body wellness.

There are distinct differences between paleo and keto but they share some characteristics. They both emphasize whole foods. This means they want you to eat foods that haven't been processed. They both get rid of legumes and grains. They may get rid of these foods for different reasons, but they both discourage them.

They both get rid of added sugars and they add in healthy fats. They are both fairly effective for losing weight.

The big difference between the two is that paleo focuses more on ideology and keto mainly focuses on macronutrients. Paleo wants people to follow the diet for lifestyle changes that help them and the environment. The keto diet doesn't have that type of philosophy. It's just a weight loss plan.

Paleo allows you to eat whole food carbs. Paleo restricts some carb sources. It's not technically a low-carb diet. Paleo also doesn't provide you any specific numbers like macronutrients that you have to follow.

The keto diet will allow you to eat some soy foods and dairy. Keto even tends to encourage the consumption of many different dairy foods like high-fat dairies such as butter, heavy cream, and unsweetened yogurt.

Milk and ice cream are prohibited on keto mainly because they don't have as much fat and are high in carbs. You can also eat soybeans, tempeh, and tofu as long as you are still able to reach you macro allotment. Soy milk though is discouraged.

Paleo does not allow soy and restricts the majority of dairy, grass-fed butter being the exception.

Both diets are okay to follow for health reasons, but the paleo diet does provide healthier options for the majority of people. It gives you more flexibility and it isn't as restrictive as keto.

Now that we've gotten that out of the way, let's dive into the ketogenic diet.

Problems with Modern Diet

Everybody is aware of the fact that obesity is on the rise. In the US, a third of all adults are obese, that's around 78.6 million. But obesity isn't the only problem. It's dangerous to the people. Obesity increases the risk of a large number of unwanted health problems such as stroke, some types of cancer, diabetes, and heart disease. In fact, it is one of the leading causes of preventable death in the United States.

Sadly, with our current modern diet, it shouldn't be surprising that society has a problem. Over the past few decades, the food that we eat and the amount of it have changed. We process our foods more, they are fried up and are placed in helpful to-go packages. They also come in super-sized portions.

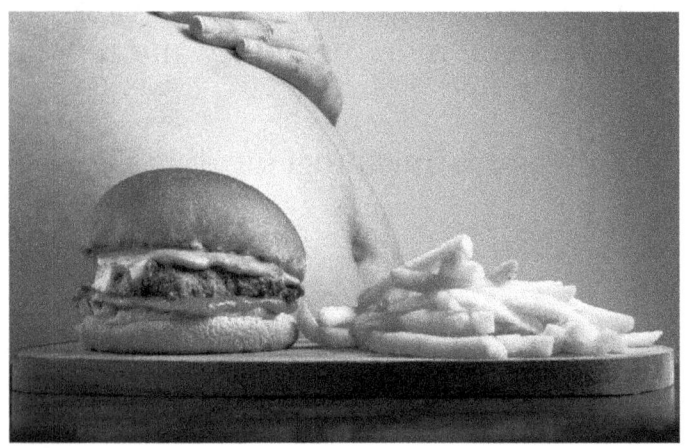

Let's have a deeper look into our modern diet and how it has affected the health of the population.

How Diet Has Changed

In just 30 to 40 years, our diet has drastically changed. Back then, the majority of the foods were fresh and grown locally. People cooked at home. Now, nearly everything that people buy is already processed, even the foods that you cook at home. This comes in the form of trans fats, sugars, colorings, chemicals, additives, and loads of other ingredients that wouldn't have been seen a couple of generations ago.

Additionally, there has been a large increase in sugar consumption over the last few decades. The average American consumes 22 teaspoons of sugar every day, or it makes up 25% of their daily calorie intake. That's an increase of 10% from just ten years ago and a 20% increase since the '70s.

The biggest cause of this is processed fructose, which is typically added to sweeten up desserts, sauces, juices, sodas, and even "healthy" drinks and meals. Kids are also eating more sugar, which is setting them up for a lifetime of poor nutrition and health.

Switching up the fats that we consume has created another problem. For a long time, people have been made to think that coconut oil, animal fats, and other healthy fats could lead to heart problems. People then substituted those fats for processed vegetable oils such as corn and canola. These oils can actually create metabolic changes and hormonal imbalances. Through the years, repeated use of these oils have perpetuated the problem with obesity and more people have turned away from the naturally-occurring, healthy, and important fats that were once used.

With the increased consumption of processed and vegetable oils, we have flooded our bodies with omega-6 fatty acids. This throws off the balance of fatty acids. When they become imbalanced, it can end up causing some types of cancer, diabetes, arthritis, Alzheimer's, and heart disease. Omega-3 fatty acids, the fats that you find in fish and fish oil, and omega-6 fatty acids need to be balanced. That means you should have one serving for every serving of the other. Today, people tend to eat around twice as many omega-6s than omega-3s.

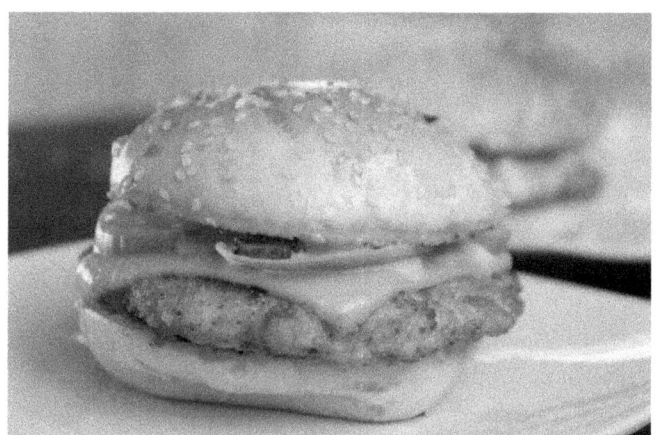

Convenience foods have also hurt our health. With the fast-paced life of society, more people eat on the go. They grab that fried, fast food that they can easily eat in the car. They grab all of those prepackaged drinks and snacks you find at the gas station. They eat meals that aren't made with natural or fresh foods. It's a trend that may be cheap and easy, but it has done more harm than good.

Back To Basics

The main key to getting our diet back where it should be is to head back to the basics. Centuries ago, cavemen weren't faced with obesity problems. Why? Because they ate foods that came from the earth, fresh fruits, vegetables, unprocessed, untouched foods, and grass-fed meats.

This is how society needs to look at food. People need to add fresh produce to every meal, and instead of staying away from fats, we need to consume good fats for our body to thrive.

The "low fat" phase during the 80s and 90s created a lot of issues for our health. Fats are important for the function of our body. In fact, for the best health, around 50 to 80 percent of our calories need to come from healthy fats. This means beans, eggs, coconut oil, olive oil, seeds, avocado, fish, and nuts. These are all found in nature.

Look At Your Diet

Take a minute to look at your current diet. What type of diet does it resemble? Is it a healthy one like the diet of a prehistoric person? Or is it a disease-riddled modern diet full of fast food? If you chose the latter, you need to make a few changes, both for your own health and your families.

The Good Parts Of The Keto Diet

Now, let me start this chapter with this. In a later chapter, we will be looking at the dangers and side effects that come along with keto diet. I choose to start with the benefits so you would understand why so many people follow the keto diet despite the downsides. So, I want you to take the good and the bad and decide for yourself if it's something you think you can do safely.

Many different things will happen when you follow a ketogenic diet. The following are just a few.

Improvement in Obesity, Metabolic Syndrome and Diabetes

This is the main reason why a lot of people follow a ketogenic diet. In all of the reasons we will look at, plus this reason, a ketogenic diet is perfect for people who suffer from type 1 or type 2 Diabetes. It is also perfect for people who are obese because it is able to help them burn off fat and it spares muscle loss. It is also able to curb a lot of disorders that tend to happen because of obesity. This includes the symptoms and risk factors known as metabolic syndrome.

Improvement in Muscle Gain and Endurance

It has been discovered that BHB helps to promote muscle gain. When you combine this with a lot of anecdotal evidence through the years, a bodybuilder movement has happened with the keto diet and how it can help them gain muscle. Ultra-endurance athletes started touse a keto diet. After an athlete has become fat-adapted, some evidence has suggested that their mental and physical performance has improved.

It Can Help the Eyes

The biggest problem that diabetics could end up facing is macular degeneration. It is common knowledge that high blood sugar can end up hurting a person's eyesight and can lead to a higher risk of cataracts. It shouldn't come as a surprise that when you lower your blood sugar levels, you will also improve your vision and eyes.

Helps Women's Health

In a 2013 review, they found that a keto diet was able to enhance fertility. They also found that PCOS could be treated effectively with a low-carb diet, which was able to reduce or completely eliminate symptoms such as infrequent or prolonged periods, obesity, and acne. Overall, when blood sugar levels are stabilized and low, it will help to equilibrate all of the other hormone levels. This is going to naturally cause a downstream effect of benefits along the metabolic pathways that are connected to insulin such as hunger and energy utilization.

Helps With Gallbladder and Gastrointestinal Health

This means that you will have less bloating and gas, improved digestion, less risk of gallstones, less acid reflux, and heartburn. It's commonly known that sugary foods, nightshades like tomatoes and potatoes, and grain-based foods increase a person's likelihood of heartburn and acid reflux. Therefore, it shouldn't come as a surprise that eating fewer carbs will improve these symptoms and confront the root problems of autoimmune responses, inflammation, and bacterial issues.

A keto diet will also reproducibly and rapidly alter the human gut microbiome. Dr. Eric Westman explains how a large number of problems are removed or reduced because of these microbiome changes. Research has also found that consuming carbs is one of the main causes of gallstones. When you consume enough fats when your carb intake is down, it will help to clear up gallbladders and make things run more smoothly.

Uric Acid Levels Will Stabilize

The biggest culprit of gout and kidney stones are high levels of uric acid, calcium, oxalate, and phosphorus. The main cause of this is typically a combination of consuming things that have a lot of alcohol and purines, unlucky genetics, dehydration, obesity, and sugar consumption. The main caveat is that a ketogenic diet can temporarily raise your uric acid levels, especially if you end up letting yourself become dehydrated. Over time, once you become adapted to the diet and you make sure you consume enough water, your levels will become lower.

Better Energy and Sleep

Once people reach day four or five of the diet, many of them report an increase in energy levels and fewer cravings for carbs. The main reason for this is again stable insulin levels and an energy source that is readily available for the brain and body tissues. It's still a mystery as to why it helps improve sleep. Studies have found that a keto diet improves sleep because it decreases REM and increases slow-wave sleep patterns. The exact reason behind this is unclear. It probably has something to do with the complex biochemical shifts involved in the brain using ketones for energy combined with body burning fat.

Lowered Inflammation

An article in *Nature Medicine* found that it was discovered that the main mechanism behind inflammation that had been believed for decades, a ketogenic diet is an anti-inflammatory diet and it can help with a lot of related issues. Research has discovered that the effects are like connected to "BHB-mediate inhibition of the NLRP3 inflammasome."

Basically, this means that inflammatory disease can be suppressed with BHB, a ketone that is produced when you follow a keto diet. This is how it caused implications concerning arthritis, IBS, acne, eczema, psoriasis, and other inflammatory diseases, and it has prompted a lot more research.

Heart Disease Prevention

A ketogenic diet is able to lower blood pressure and triglyceride level and improve your cholesterol profiles. The reason for this is because of the effects of keeping blood glucose at a low and stable level. While it will likely sound counterintuitive that consuming more fat is going to reduce your triglycerides, it has been discovered that too many carbs are the main reason for high triglyceride levels. When you look at HDL and LDL levels, a keto diet can help to raise your good cholesterol and to lower your bad cholesterol.

Can Fight off Cancer

Dom D'Agostino's lab found that ketone supplementation is able to decrease the viability of tumor cells and prolonged the life of mice that had metastatic cancer. Cancer cell metabolism works abnormally compared to healthy cells. They increase through glucose consumption because of mitochondrial dysfunction and genetic mutations. Some studies have found that unlike healthy tissues, cancer cells can't effectively use ketone bodies for energy. Ketones will also inhibit the viability and proliferation of tumor cells. This doesn't mean a cancer patient should forgo regular treatment. You should still follow your doctor's advice.

Improves the Brain's Focus

The ketogenic diet can help increase memory, clarity, cognition, seizure control, and fewer migraines. The first notable use of the keto diet was in the 1920s at the Mayo Clinic to help children with epilepsy. While the exact reason behind seizure prevention on a keto diet is still unknown, scientists think it's because it causes an increased stability of neurons and upregulation of mitochondrial enzymes and brain mitochondria.

Similar to this, there is a lot of attention given to this diet and its effects on Alzheimer's disease. Researchers have found that there is an increase in cognition and improved memory in adults with problems in these areas, and more research has found improvement in all dementia stages. Ketosis is also able to help fight Parkinson's disease.

For the wider audience of keto diet followers, there are reported side effects of fewer intense and less frequent migraines and better mental focus and clarity. This is likely due to more stable blood sugar and change in brain chemistry that helps cognition and memory too.

Getting Started with Keto

The terms ketogenic and keto can be used interchangeably as you have probably already noticed. The word keto was derived from the fact that when following this type of diet, your body will create small fuel molecules which are called ketones. Your body will use these as an alternative fuel source, which gets used after your body's stored glucose is depleted.

Once you start eating fewer carbs, ketones will be produced. This will remain true as long as your protein intake is kept at a moderate level. Too much protein is able to be switched into sugar just like carbs.

Ketones are created by the liver from the fat stores in your body. The body will then consume these ketones as a fuel source throughout the different areas in your body and the brain. The brain uses way more energy throughout the day than any other part of your body, but it can't run off of fat. The only fuel source that works for the brain is glucose or ketones.

When it comes to following a keto diet, the entire body will switch its fuel supply so that it can run almost completely on fat. This means that your insulin levels are going to drop and you will increase how much fat you burn. Your body will discover that it is easier to access your stored fat and burn them. This is a great byproduct of the keto diet when you are trying to lose some weight, but there are many other less obvious benefits such as mental alertness, lower hunger levels, and steadier energy.

How Low is Low?

The only way that a keto diet will work for you is if you consume very little carbs. The fewer the carbs you eat, the better it will be when it comes to losing weight. This makes the keto diet an extremely strict low-carb diet. The majority of people are only allowed to consume 20 grams or less of net carbs per day. After you have reached your ideal weight, you can then start to increase the carbs you eat. This needs to be done very slowly in order to make sure that you don't gain back the weight you lost.

First Things First

While this is a pretty effective weight loss diet, there is a right and a wrong way to do it. You need to make sure that you start off the right way in order to ensure that you get the best and fastest results.

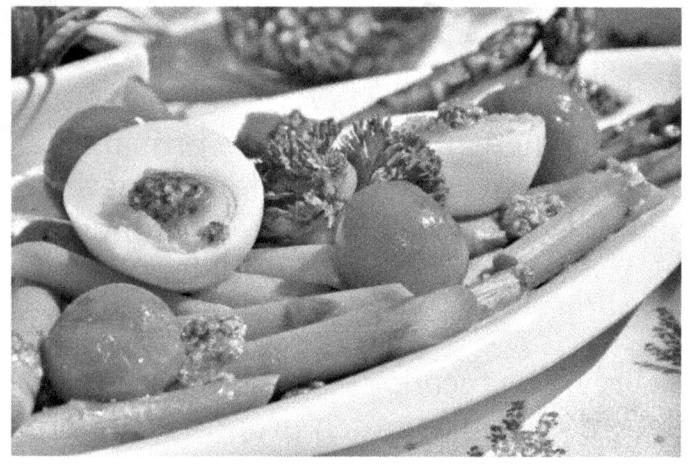

In theory, a ketogenic diet is pretty simple. You eat low amounts of carbs and high amounts of fat. But in practice, it's a bit more complicated. You need to know what you can and cannot eat. In a later chapter, you will find a more complete list of the things that you can and can't eat, but let's have a look at a basic list of these foods.

- Heavy fats such as olive oil, bacon fat, tallow, lard, ghee, butter, and coconut oil.
- Meats and that include organ meats as well.
- Eggs
- Seafood and fish.
- Non-starchy vegetables. You will definitely want leafy greens.
- Some berries, like blueberries, strawberries, and raspberries.

This means that a typical day could look like:

- Breakfast: bacon and eggs.
- Lunch: chicken salad with a cup of bone broth.
- Dinner: steak with a side of veggies and a ketogenic dessert.

There are some people who will eat a snack in between their meals. There isn't any need for a snack unless you need a little energy boost or are feeling a bit hungry. Some good snack ideas are meat sticks, celery sticks, nuts, broth, and cheese sticks. You have to keep an eye on your snacks though, they will add to your complete macro count.

You can also easily personalize the keto diet. You have the power to experiment with things to see what is going to work best for you. There are some people who discover that they need to eat more fats while other people are able to eat a lot fewer carbs. Some people even use intermittent fasting.

The majority of those people who choose to follow intermittent fasting will skip breakfast and eat their first meal at one. This will raise their ketosis. There are a lot of people who find that they naturally fall into intermittent fasting because they don't feel as hungry. And that's fine too.

Macronutrients

Macros have already been mentioned several times in this book and you are probably ready to learn more about them. Macro is a short-term for macronutrients when you are talking about a ketogenic diet.

Macros are the different parts of the food that you eat which provides you with energy and fuel. The three macros are protein, fat, and carbohydrates. These are the areas where all of your dietary calories are going to come from. This is probably the biggest thing that you really need to learn in order to make sure that you are successful with the keto diet. You need to make sure that they stay in the right balance in order to ensure that you remain in ketosis.

Carbohydrates are the only macro that you don't have to consume in order to survive. There are essential amino acids and fatty acids which are the building blocks of proteins and fats, but there aren't any essential carbohydrates.

Carbs are made up of two things, starches and sugars. Fiber is viewed as a carb, but with a keto diet, it isn't counted towards a total carb intake. The reason fiber isn't counted is that the body doesn't really digest fiber, so it doesn't have much of an effect on your blood sugar.

This means, when you pick up something and read its nutritional label, the first thing that you need to look at is the total carbs. Then have a look at the dietary fiber. After that, you will need to subtract the amount of fiber content from the total carb amount. This is going to give you what is known as net carb content.

It looks like this:

Total carbs – fiber = net carbs

This makes sure that the only carbs that are counted are the starches and the sugars in each of the carbohydrates. When you have to figure out the macros in a meal, you will only have to look at the net carbs and you don't have to look at the complete carbs. Now, there are some foods that don't contain any dietary fiber, and in that case, you would use the complete carb amount.

In order to make sure that you succeed, you will need to figure out the foods that are naturally low in carbs and the ones that are not. Not all of these foods sources will be obvious. Everybody knows potatoes are high in carbs, they are starchy, but did you realize that bananas are also high in carbs?

Before we get into the nitty gritty of figuring out your macro numbers, a basic rule of them is that you shouldn't consume more than 20 grams of net carbs every day.

It's crucial that you consume enough protein because it is important for the body. It helps to preserve your lean muscle mass, it's an energy source when there aren't any carbs, it creates enzymes and hormones, it helps the immune function, repairs tissue, and helps it grow. The biological process requires protein. Proteins are the building blocks for a healthy body.

When you eat proteins, your body will break them down into amino acids. Nine of the amino acids that protein produces are cannot be produced by the body alone. This is the reason why these essential amino acids must come from the foods you eat. These nine amino acids are valine, tryptophan, threonine, phenylalanine, methionine, lysine, leucine, isoleucine, and histidine. When you have protein deficiency or a deficiency in any of these amino acids, it can end up causing malnutrition, kwashiorkor, or a whole host of other health problems.

When you follow a ketogenic diet, it's imperative that you make sure that you eat enough protein in order to preserve your lean body mass. The amount that you consume will greatly depend on how much lean body mass you currently have. Here is a guideline.

- .7 to .8 grams of protein per pound of muscle to help preserve your muscle mass.

- .8 to 1.2 grams of protein per pound of muscle to help you increase your muscle mass.

Your goal should never be to lose body mass. You should only want to preserve or gain it. There are a lot of people that are focused on losing weight, but there are times that losing weight will cause you to lose muscle along with fat. Your goal should be to lose fat and save your muscle. This plays an important role in making sure that you keep a good metabolism.

The main thing you need to remember is that you shouldn't go overly crazy when eating protein on a ketogenic diet. Too much protein could end up stressing your kidneys too much and it could affect your level of ketosis. As long as you keep your macros in the appropriate range, all should be okay.

Here is a great example to go by.

Let's assume that you weigh 160 pounds and you have 30 percent body fat. This means you have around 48 pounds of body fat. Then you can subtract your body fat from your total weight. This will give you your lean body mass. For this example, it would be 112 pounds.

To figure out how much protein you should consume, you have to take the lean body mass number and multiply by the ratio from earlier. For this example, you would have to consume 89.6 grams of protein each day to preserve your muscle mass. The computation looks like this.

112 pounds muscle x .8 grams protein = 89.6 grams

The macro we need to go over is fat. Fat needs to be consumed in adequate amounts in order for your body to maintain cell membranes, provide protective cushioning for organs, absorb certain vitamins, development, growth, and energy. With the keto diet, fats also help you to stay full.

In the body, dietary fat is broken into glycerol and fatty acids. The body isn't able to synthesize two types of fatty acids, so you have to make sure that you consume them in your regular diet. These include linoleic acid and linolenic acid.

These fats are sating, so it's perfect for people looking to fight off hunger pangs. Now you have to figure out how much fat you need to eat. If your carbs are at a minimum, you've figured out how much protein you need to eat, and then the rest of your dietary needs have to be met with fat.

To maintain weight, you will eat enough calories from fat to support your regular expenditure. If you want to burn fat, then you will have to eat in a deficit.

Now, I have given you a lot of information to help you figure out your macros. However, there is a lot easier way to figure this out. There are a lot of online calculators to figure out these numbers without getting a headache. If you want to use an online calculator, check out the website Ketogains. They have one that works great.

Now, if you want to see how figuring it out on your own will work, let's continue with the 160-pound example from earlier. Let's say this person is a female, stands 5'4", in her late 20s, and has a desk job. She's mainly sedentary.

Plugging in her info into a calculator:

The base metabolic rate would be 1467 kcal.

Daily energy expenditure would be 1614 kcal.

She would need to eat around 90 grams of protein, 20 grams of net carbs, and 86 grams of fat. Her intake is made up of 72 percent fat, 23 percent protein, and 5 percent carbs.

Now you know what macros are and how to figure out your numbers. You are well on your way to getting started with a ketogenic diet.

The Problems With Keto

While for the most part, the ketogenic diet is a safe and effective diet, it does come with some dangers and sides effects. Before we go into the dangers of keto, let's look at the most common side effects that you could end up experiencing once your body enters ketosis.

Side Effects

Not all of the side effects of the ketogenic diet are bad, but there are going to be some unpleasant ones that you may experience.

1. Very little energy.

This is a very common problem when your body is starting to adjust to your new source of energy. Luckily, after your body has adjusted to using fat as energy, your energy will go up.

2. You A1C levels could improve.

If you are diabetic, the better blood sugar control could help to control your A1C and it might even reduce your need for insulin. That doesn't mean you should go off your meds though. The only caveat is that it does also increase your risk of diabetic ketoacidosis, which is life-threatening. This is more common for people with type 1 diabetes, but if you have type 2, you should still talk to your doctor first.

3. You won't have as much brain fog.

It is a well-known fact that carbs, especially the refined kinds like white pasta, white bread, and sugar will end up causing your blood sugar to spike and then dip. So it's very easy to see why when you eat fewer carbs, you will be able to keep your blood sugar levels steady. For healthy people, this means that they will keep a steady energy level, less brain fog, and fewer sugar cravings.

4. You may notice that your skin clears up.

If you have been bothered by pimples, you could find that the keto diet could clear them up. This is especially true if you used to be a sugar addict. Empty carbs are the worst thing for acne because they trigger inflammation. Some studies have found that curbing your carb intake could fix those types of problems.

5. You will have increased thirst.

You shouldn't worry if you start to notice that you feel more parched when you start your keto diet. Your body is going to be excreting a lot more water and this will make you thirsty. The important thing is to remember that you drink plenty of water.

There is no exact amount that you have to drink, but you should make sure that you drink enough water to turn your urine clear to pale yellow.

6. You may notice that you are feeling less hungry.

Most diets are associated with fighting off cravings and feeling hungry. That's not necessarily the case with the keto diet. There are a lot of people who report less hunger and a diminished need for eating. Researchers aren't completely sure why this happens, but it's believed that low carb diets suppress the hormone ghrelin which controls hunger.

7. Your weight will likely drop quickly, but you may notice that some come back.

The reason the ketogenic diet became so popular is that of its initial quick slim down. The reason for this is because your body will release quite a bit of water when you switch to using fat as energy. The scales will likely show that you have lost a few pounds and you could even look leaner.

That first drop in weight that you notice is likely going to be just water weight. This doesn't mean that you've not burned off fat. The problem comes with the fact that while studies have discovered that you will lose weight, they have yet to figure out if it can be sustained. Most people will find that this type of strict diet is hard to stick to. If you do veer off of your diet, you could find that you gain some of the weight back.

8. You can end up feeling sick and tired.

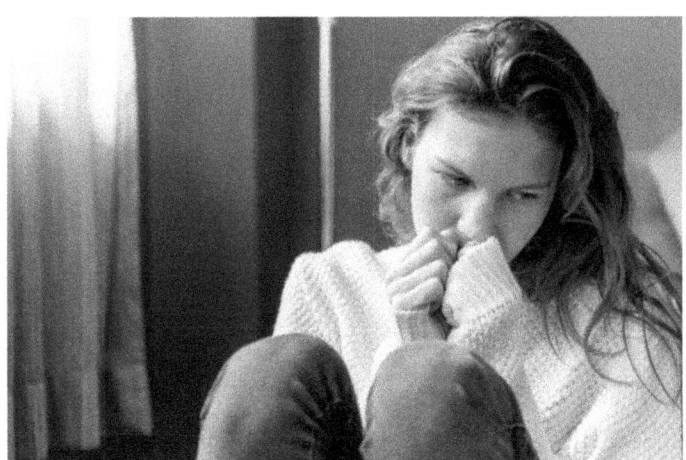

The keto flu is completely real. When you cut your carbs and reach ketosis, it will bring about a number of uncomfortable symptoms such as diarrhea, nausea, muscle aches, fatigue, and headaches. These side effects are caused by the body transitioning into using fat as its main energy source instead of carbs. Once your body has adapted to this fuel source in about a week or two, you will notice that you feel a lot better.

The Dangers of Keto

Now, we've talked through some of the side effects that you could experience until your body gets used in using fat as a fuel source. The negative side effects will go away. The following things that could happen when following a keto diet may not.

These are all rare things and typically will only happen if you don't eat healthily and follow your macros, but it could end up happening. It's important to know them so that you can avoid them.

1. Cardiac Issues

Losing some heart muscle isn't the only heart-associated risk that could come along with the keto diet. If you are already on medication for high blood pressure and you are on the keto diet, you could end up with abnormally low blood pressure results. If you already have a heart condition, talk to your doctor before you start a keto diet.

2. Muscle Loss

The longer you allow your body to stay in ketosis, the more fat it is going to burn. But you could cause your body to start burning off muscle tissue too. While consuming enough protein does wonders for building up muscle, your muscles can also use carbs for their formation and maintenance. Without consuming carbs, your body could possibly start breaking down its own muscles.

3. Kidney Damage and Stones

If you do let yourself get dehydrated and you don't take control of it quickly, it could end up causing acute kidney injury. But this isn't the only way that it could cause damage to your kidneys. Too much protein can end up creating high nitrogen levels which will cause the pressure in your kidneys to increase. This may end up creating kidney stones that can end up hurting your kidney cells.

4. Dehydration

This is a very common thing for people who are just starting the keto diet because ketosis will cause your body to flush out excess water. In order to prevent dehydration, you should try to aim for 2.5 liters of water every day. You need to start drinking this much water as soon as you start a ketogenic diet. You do not need to wait until you start noticing the side effects of dehydration.

5. Decreased Serum Sodium

Most Americans will consume too much salt, but for a person that is following a ketogenic diet, they can sometimes struggle to consume enough. Low sodium levels can end up causing confusion, leg cramps, decreased energy, and vomiting. Make sure that all of your meals have salt added to them. Sea salt is the best choice because it also contains trace minerals.

6. Loss of Electrolytes

When you hit ketosis, your body will start to dump stores of glycogen which is found in your muscles and fat that carries extra weight. This will make you use the bathroom more and will lead to electrolyte loss. Electrolytes are important for proper cardiac function and normal heartbeats. This could cause a cardiac arrhythmia. Try to get more electrolytes through natural sources or through OTC supplements.

7. Bowel Changes and Constipation

Besides not getting their nutrients, eliminating veggies and fruits causes other problems as well. They are fiber-rich foods that help keep you regular. Without those foods, you may find that you start having bowel changes which include difficulty in bowel movements and possible constipation.

You will need to make sure you load up on fiber-rich, low-carb foods like cabbage, asparagus, and broccoli, as well as more fats like ghee and coconut oil.

8. Nutritional Deficiencies

A high-fat, low-carb diet will limit the kinds of foods that you are able to eat and complete food groups will be eliminated. Whole grains, beans, and legumes are all out, and so are a lot of vegetables and fruits. Most of the foods carry nutrients, vitamins, and minerals that you aren't able to get anywhere else. Without those foods, you could end up experiencing nutritional deficiencies.

Keto isn't good for a long-term diet because it's not balanced. Diets that are devoid of veggies and fruits will cause long-term micronutrient deficiencies that will come along with other consequences. It's great for short-term fat loss, but it is best under the supervision of a medical professional.

9. Low Blood Sugar

For the most part, once you have reached ketosis, you will notice more stable and lower blood sugar levels. That's why low-carb diets are effective at controlling type 2 diabetes. Carb monitoring has been used for a while now as a way to control blood sugar. But one study has found that low-carb diets aren't better for long-term control than any other diet.

There is some anecdotal evidence that says people with type 2 diabetes were able to stop taking their medicine because they were about to stabilize their blood sugar. But that is in no way recommended and people with diabetes must talk to their doctor first.

Those first few days while the body is adapting to the changes, your body is in a constant struggle. You will need to ease your way into the diet if you have diabetes. Slowly cut back on your carbs, otherwise, you could cause your blood sugar to drop too much.

Ketosis and How to Reach It

We've talked about ketosis a lot. We've even talked about what it does to the body. There is still a lot about ketosis that you have yet to learn, like how to get into it and what it means to your health. Let's look even further into what it is. The important thing to know is that ketosis is a natural state that your body will enter when it is being fueled by fat. This can happen if a person fasts or if they follow a very strict low-carb diet.

There are many different benefits for ketosis like performance, health, and weight loss. But like what we talked in the last chapter, it also comes along with some unpleasant side effects. For people who have type 1 diabetes and certain other disease types, too many ketones in their body can end up becoming dangerous.

Once your body enters ketosis, it will start to produce ketones. Ketones are small fuel molecules and the body will use them as an alternative source of energy once your glucose stores have been depleted. The liver will change your fat into ketones that are then sent into the blood. The body will then use the ketones just like it used glucose. Ketones can also fuel the brain.

Reaching Ketosis

There are two ways for your body to reach ketosis: A Ketogenic diet or fasting. Under either one of these circumstances, once the body's limited amount of glucose has been depleted, the body will switch its source for fuel to fat. The fat-storing hormone, insulin, will become low, and the body's fat burning will be increased. This means that your body has easy access to your fats stores and can get rid of them.

You are considered to be in ketosis once your body produces enough ketones to make a significant level in the blood, usually more than .5mm. The quickest way for this to happen is through fasting, but it isn't something you can do forever. That is why people turn to a keto diet because it can be eaten for an indefinite amount of time.

Fuel for the Brain

A lot of people think you have to have carbs to fuel your brain. The brain will happily burn carbs when you consume them, but when carbs aren't available it will happily eat ketones.

This is necessary for basic survival. Since the body is only able to store carbs for a day or two, the brain would end up shutting down after a few days with no food. Alternatively, it would need to quickly convert muscle protein into glucose, which isn't very efficient just in order to keep working. That would mean we could waste away very quickly. If this was the way the body worked, then the human race wouldn't have been able to survive before 24/7 food became available.

The body has evolved to work smarter than that. Normally, the body will have fat stores that will last so that a person can survive for several weeks without food. Ketosis is the process that happens to make sure that the brain is able to run on those fat stores.

How to Reach Optimal Ketosis

This is what everybody on a ketogenic diet wants. When you reach optimal ketosis, your body will burn fat at the most optimal speed. To reach this optimal ketosis, you have to follow the low-carb, high-fat diet as laid out above, keeping your macros in the optimal range. There isn't any trick to help you reach this optimal level. There are some things you can do.

Here are the different ketone levels you could have.

- Below 0.5 means that you are not in ketosis.
- Between 0.5 and 1.5 is a light level of nutritional ketosis. You will be losing weight, but it won't be optimal.
- Around 1.5 to 3 is what is considered optimal ketosis and is best for maximum weight loss.
- Levels over 3 aren't needed. High levels aren't going to help you one way or the other and could end up harming you because it could mean that you aren't getting enough food.

There are a lot of people who believe that they are consuming a strict keto diet but end up being surprised when they measure their blood ketone levels. When measured, they end up being around 0.2 or 0.5, which isn't at that sweet spot.

The trick to get past this plateau is that you not only have to avoid the obvious carb sources but making sure your protein intake doesn't get higher than your fat intake. I know I said protein won't affect your glucose levels as easily as carbs do, but if you consume too many, especially if you eat more than fat, it will affect your glucose. This will compromise your optimal ketosis.

The secret to working around this problem is to increase your intake of fat. You can do this by adding a big dollop of herbed butter to your steak. This could keep you from eating as much or going back for seconds.

Having a glass of bulletproof coffee can also help to stave off hunger and prevents you from eating as much protein. This is as simple as adding a tablespoon of butter and a tablespoon of coconut oil to your coffee in the morning.

The more fats you eat, the fuller you will feel. This will make sure that you don't eat too much protein and you will eat fewer carbohydrates. This should help you to reach optimal ketosis.

How to Measure Ketosis

There are a few ways to figure out whether or not you have reached ketosis. The first way is measuring ketones in your blood. This requires purchasing a meter and will require a prick on the finger.

There are quite a few reasonably priced gadgets out there for this, and it only takes a few seconds to find out what your blood ketone level is. Most people don't go to this extreme to find out what their ketone level is, but it is the most accurate and effective.

You should measure your blood ketones first thing in the morning and on a fasted stomach. You can follow the levels that I listed earlier in this chapter to figure out if you are in ketosis.

These meters measure the amount of BHB that you have in your blood. This is the main ketone that will be present when in ketosis. The main downside of using this method is the fact that you have to draw blood.

Finding a test kit will cost around $30 to $40, and could cost an extra $5 for every test. This is the reason why those who choose to test this way will only perform one test every week or every other week.

All right, so if you don't want to go to the expense of getting a blood ketone meter, we've got six other options to figure out whether or not you are in ketosis.

1. Bad breath

This doesn't sound pleasant but people will often say they have bad breath when they hit ketosis. This is a fairly common side effect. People will often say that their breath becomes fruitier.

The reason for this is the elevated ketone levels. The main culprit is the ketone acetone that the body excretes through your breath and urine. While you may not like the idea of having bad breath, it is a great way to know you're in ketosis. A lot of people will brush their teeth more often or chew sugar-free gum.

2. Ketones in urine and breath

If you don't want to prick your finger, you can measure blood ketones with a breath analyzer. This will monitor for acetone which is one of the three ketones that will be present in your blood once you reach ketosis.

This will let you know when your ketone levels have hit ketosis level because acetone will only leave the body once you reach nutritional ketosis. These breath analyzers are fairly accurate, though not as accurate as a blood monitor.

Another way to check for ketosis is to check for ketones in the urine every day using special indicator strips. This is a quick and cheap method to use to assess what your ketone levels are everyday. These aren't the most reliable methods though.

3. Better energy and focus

A lot of people will sometimes report feeling sick, tired, or have brain fog once they first start a keto diet. This is the keto flu, but people who follow this long-term will report better energy and increased focus. Your body has to take the time to adapt to the new diet. Once you hit ketosis, your brain will start burning ketones for energy and this could take a week or so to start happening.

Ketones are a more potent fuel source for the brain as opposed to carbs. This means that it will improve your mental clarity and brain function.

4. Short-term performance decrease

Just like with number three, the fatigue can cause a decrease in exercise performance. This is due to the reduction in your muscle glycogen stores, which is what typically provides you with the fuel you need for high-intensity exercises. After a week or so your performance levels should return to normal.

5. Digestive issues

With the major changes to the foods you eat, you will probably experience diarrhea or constipation in the beginning. This lets you know that you are reaching ketosis. After your transition period, these issues should go away.

6. Insomnia

One of the biggest issues a keto dieter will have is insomnia especially when they first start. When a person's carbs are drastically reduced, it can cause sleeping issues. However, this too shall pass.

There are a lot of different signs and symptoms that will let you know if you are in ketosis and if you are doing things correctly. Ultimately, if you follow the rules for a keto diet and you keep yourself consistent, your body will be in some form of ketosis.

If you want to know absolutely for certain whether or not you are in ketosis, the only way to do that is with a blood ketone monitor.

Making Keto Work For Everybody

Most people will stay away from diets if they think they are too hard to put into their lives. The great thing about the keto diet is, it isn't that hard to implement and it shouldn't interfere with your life in any way. To help everyone feel like they can follow a keto diet, this chapter will look at eating on a budget, eating out, eating during the holiday, and even more.

Keto on a Budget

Many people assume that eating keto will be expensive, but it really isn't. Your fat intake is going to be upped. Fats help make you feel fuller than carbs will. This means that you can go longer between meals. Not eating snacks all the time will help you save money too.

Since protein levels aren't really going to change, you aren't going to be faced with having to buy expensive meats. Here are some money-saving tips.

- Keep things simple. Your meals don't have to be difficult and have many different parts. The fewer ingredients you use, the less money you are going to spend. If you make a simple omelet and drink water, it is going to cost you about $3.50. A Big Mac will cost you $5.
- You get a better deal if you buy a whole chicken and cut it up yourself. Keep the bones too. You can use it to make broth.
- Buy fresh vegetables when they are in season. The rest of the year, you can purchase frozen.
- Watch for sales at your grocery store. Stock up on these items especially if you use a lot of them.

It also helps if you can plan out your meal in advance and make a shopping list. This will ensure you stay organized. You will just buy what you need. Planning your shopping list is the best way to stop all unnecessary spending and impulse buying.

While shopping, here are some things you can do to save money.

- Purchase regular cheese. There is no reason to purchase the expensive specialty cheeses. Buy in bulk if you can, and never purchase pre-shredded. Find a block of cheese and shred it yourself.
- Just like cheese, buy simple meats and avoid specialty ones. Cooked meats make a fast meal but choose the less exotic types.

- Don't buy the bags of coleslaw. Buy a head of cabbage and shred it yourself. It will last longer and you will get more meals out of it.

- Don't worry about finding kale. Find other leafy greens that are cheaper and just as nutritious.

- Only buy avocados when they are in season.

- Stop buying nuts because these get expensive, especially macadamias.

- Get an almond meal instead of almond flour. It is cheaper and works as well as almond flour in recipes. You could also grind your own almonds.

- Buy frozen or canned fish instead of fresh, especially when talking about salmon.

Get the best quality foods that you can afford. Just because everyone says you need to eat organic doesn't mean you absolutely have to. If you can't afford something, then don't get it. The important thing is that you make your meals at home from scratch. They will be healthier even if they aren't organic.

When choosing meats, go with a cheaper cut and make sure you look for bargains or reduced meats.

You need to cook all of your meals at home. This is cheaper and healthier than eating out. Go with easy recipes and avoid all the fancy keto recipes.

Traveling

The most important part of any diet is maintaining it when you aren't at home. The key to making sure you maintain your diet is planning. The following will help you maintain your diet while you are traveling.

- Know your macros

Before taking a vacation, you need to know what your macros are. Make sure you have them memorized or have a keto app on your phone that helps track your macros.

- Food options

You must think about the foods you can take. Non-perishable foods are the best options. Canned salmon, tuna, chicken, and beef jerky are all great options. Canned shakes and olives are also great to take with you. All of your snacks like string cheese, pepperoni, and dried nuts are also great. If you like eating eggs, hard boil them to take them along.

When talking about foods that need refrigeration, if you aren't traveling too far from home, you should purchase any perishables when you have arrived. This is where it is important to have a refrigerator at the place you are staying.

Once you arrive, go to the store and buy your cheese and meats. One other option is making your meals ahead of time and freezing them before a trip. Pack them in a cooler and put them in the freezer once you arrive. Every morning, set the meals for that day in the refrigerator to thaw.

- Travel evaluation

You need to know how long your trip is going to take. If it is just overnight, it is going to be fairly easy to prepare. You just need a few frozen meals, a microwave, and a cooler. If your trip is going to be all week, it does change things and create complications. You have to know what you are going to be up against.

Once you have your location and length of your trip, begin to look at resources that will be available to you when you get there.

It is good to book a place that has a kitchen in it like an Airbnb. If you are staying at a hotel, find a room at an extended-stay hotel. These places have better cooking equipment than normal motels and hotels. This increases your flexibility when prepping meals. It would be great if you could find a place that has a full-size refrigerator and freezer. Staying with family and friends is good since you would have access to a full kitchen.

How you get to your destination is important too. If you are driving, you have more flexibility than traveling by plane. TSA restrictions might prevent you from bringing specific foods with you because they need to be repacked and weigh less than three ounces.

- Restaurants

Many restaurants and fast food places offer low carb options now. If you want a burger, just ask them to wrap it in a lettuce leaf or just leave off the bun. Choosing meats like steak and fish will keep you on your low-carb diet. Never order fries or potatoes. Stay away from rice and beans. Instead, order roasted vegetables, asparagus, and salads. If there is a Chipotle near you, you can get a bowl without bean or rice and fill it with guacamole, sour cream, cheese, and meat.

Traveling doesn't mean you have to stop your diet. There are many ways to work around this. It really isn't that hard if you plan ahead.

Keto While Dining Out

Have you been asked out by friends? Are you afraid to go? You don't have to be. You can eat delicious foods no matter where you go.

- Avoid starches

Stay away from bread. Say no to pasta. Pass on the potatoes. Bounce the rice. Never put temptations on your plate. Make sure you order meals without starchy sides.

When ordering an entrée, most places let you substitute the starchy sides for more vegetables or a salad. When you order a sandwich or burger, ask for it to be wrapped in lettuce instead. If they won't make any changes, just don't order it.

When you get your plate and it has a starch on it, look at the options. If you can leave it there and not eat it, go for it. If you can't handle the temptation, ask the server to replace it to get rid of the starch. If the restaurant is casual, you can take care of things by just throwing it away.

- Be careful with condiments and sauces

Sauces like Bearnaise sauce contain mostly fats. Ketchup contains many carbs. Gravies might end up going either way. If you aren't sure about a particular sauce, ask what's in it and stay away if it has sugar or flour in it. You could also ask if they would place the sauce on the side so you could choose whether or not to eat it.

- Add good fats

Restaurant meals are usually low in fats. This makes it hard for us to feel full when not eating carbs. You can change this inmany different ways. Ask for extra butter and put it on your vegetables or meats. Choose a vinegar and olive oil based dressing for your salad. Many restaurants serve cheap vegetable oils that are full of Omega 6 fatty acids instead of olive oil. An advanced keto dieter will carry a small bottle of olive oil with them.

- Choose drinks wisely

The best choices would be sparkling water, unsweetened tea, coffee, and water. If you want an alcoholic beverage, choose a dry wine, champagne, or spirits, either straight or with club soda.

- Dessert

If you aren't hungry, have a cup of coffee to finish off your meal. If you still feel a bit hungry, see if they have a cheese plate or some berries and whipped cream.

- Buffets

This is when things can get tricky. Set ground rules before you leave the table. Stay away from all grains and starches and aim for proteins, vegetables, and fats. Find the smallest plate and go back for more if the first plate doesn't fill you up. Be sure you take your time eating. Talk with friends and sip on your drink.

Keto and the Holidays

Holidays are always going to happen. These are the hardest times of the year to stay on any diet. This is the time to sit on the couch, eat too much, and watch too much television. This is fine, but this doesn't mean you have to stop doing keto. It is during these times when you need to reevaluate yourself and check on your keto lifestyle. Take a look at the progress you've made already and learn how to move past these anxiety-inducing moments. Here's how.

1. Keep a Keto Positive Mind

What does it mean to have a keto positive mind? Look at it like the Commandments of the Low Carb Followers. Thou shalt not drool over thy neighbor's turkey sandwich, thou shalt not make friends feel bad for having fries, thou shalt not gloat, and so on. You, you are doing keto, but you are also a compassionate and an awesome person too. Keep yourself composed and stay on keto.

2. Knowledge is Power

There are tons of apps out there that you can download for free that lets you know what is in the food you are about to eat. This means, if you see some cheese making its rounds at a party, you don't have to feel bad for tasting it. The trick to succeeding during the holidays is knowing what to say yes to and by making smart decisions. MyFitnessPal is a great choice to keep track of meals and figuring out what is in your food.

3. Create Clear Goals

The best way to make sure that you stay on track is to come up with clear goals. Everybody's keto lifestyle is a little bit different. The rules you come up will need to be based on what your goals are, which will end up determining your actions. If you're looking to drop excess fat, that's going to look different than somebody that is trying maintain or gain. A keto-warrior could have a five-point backup plan. The best goals are your own goals.

4. Plan to Fail

What does it mean to plan to fail? This means you set the bar so high that even if you don't reach your goal, you still have done better than your expectations. This is the best win-win situation. It's also very easy to do. If you know desserts are your weakness, make your own keto cheesecake and take it to the party. Now you can have your cake and eat it too.

5. Never Engage in a Debate

When you get into the keto lifestyle, you might find it tempting to try to convert others to your way of life. But it's important to understand that not everybody wants to take that step, especially when it comes to the holidays. Your aunt may not understand the reason why you have bacon for every meal of the day and nor does she want to. The important thing is to make sure you are taking the steps you need to in order to stay on track. You don't have to look out for the entire family.

6. Plan Things Away from the Couch or Table

One easy way to stay keto is to change how you see everything. Instead of waiting for people to invite you to a party, where you end up anxious about what foods they will have, make the plans yourself. Invite your family and friends on a trip, a walk around town, or to see a show. There are a lot of free events around the holidays and everybody will feel happier with some exercise.

7. Be Gracious and Have an Escape

This brings us to another point, the holidays tend to be hard for everybody. There's lots of traveling, lots of families and everybody has to make sacrifices. That could mean you have to chock down your mom's over-seasoned meatloaf, but do it with a smile on your face because it's the holidays. A small sacrifice isn't going to be a big deal when you look at the grander scheme of things. You could also try to keep from visiting around mealtimes.

8. Cheating is Fine, Just Set Some Rules

A huge taboo for keto land is cheating. When somebody breaks the rules and eats something that they regret, they end up sitting around lambasting their self for weeks on end. Stop it. You are in charge of the rules and you can change those rules. If you have a round of fries, it doesn't mean you have screwed everything up. Don't take these slips so hard and it will be easier to get back on track.

9. Remain Calm

The holidays only come around once every year, but you have keto for the rest of your life. If you have to take a few weeks off and enjoy all the great festivities, go ahead. If you feel like you need to up your gym time to make up for some carb eating, do it. If you are a keto warrior, then keto on. Nobody is going to judge you for trying to do your best during the craziest time of year. Don't kill yourself over having too many cookies, or that cup of apple cider. Just get back on track and everything is going to be fine.

10. Say Thank You

You are going to be offered all sorts of things. It's what happens during the holidays. The best thing to do is say thank you, accept it, and continue to talk. Odds are, they won't even notice that you didn't eat their fudge. If you tell them no, it might upset them. Repeat after me, "Awesome, thank you," take it and smile.

Is Keto A Good Fit?

The keto diet gets a lot of praises for being a wonderful weight loss plan. This high-fat, low-carb life might not be right for you.

You might have read some articles about this diet already. It might sound just like any other fad diet that won't last. Truth is, this diet has been around for over 100 years. This diet has many health benefits. Research has shown us this diet can help lose weight, prevent obesity, improve alertness and cognition, improve metabolic and cardiovascular conditions, and treat epilepsy.

This happens when you get into ketosis. Our bodies go through various phases of hormonal and metabolic adaptations so it learns how to use the new source of energy it is getting from fat.

When our bodies don't have glucose available for fuel, these fatty acids will get turned into ketones that go across the blood-brain barrier that will give the heart, muscles, and brain more energy. It minimizes all the excess fat that has been stored in our bodies.

Just like any diet, there are some safety problems that you have to keep in mind. The keto diet isn't right for every person. Here are some situations where the keto diet might be dangerous and you should avoid it.

Nursing or Pregnant

There haven't been many studies done to figure out all the side effects of the keto diet on pregnant women. Studies have shown some of the side effects may include constipation, anemia, inadequate growth in children, hormonal changes, nutrient deficiency, dehydration, and weight loss.

Prolonged ketosis when pregnant can cause developmental problems with the baby that can affect how well their brains develop and increase the risk of birth defects such as spina bifida.

Because of all the risk of possible harm to the baby, doctors do not recommend this diet to pregnant women.

Just like with pregnant women, there haven't been many studies done about the keto diet and nursing women. Many women who are either nursing or pregnant need more protein and fiber than women who are not pregnant or nursing. The increased fiber helps to support fetal development and growth. It helps improve the mom's digestion and gives both mom and the baby the minerals and vitamins they need.

Because we don't really know the exact results of a keto diet on moms who are nursing, it is best to adopt a moderate carb intake that keeps both mom and the baby safe.

Medicines That Could Cause Hypoglycemia

These medicines can cause hypoglycemia.

- Sulphonylureas like glipizide, tolbutamide, gliclazide, glimepiride, and glibenclamide
- Glinides like repaglinide or nateglinide
- Insulin

These medicines were designed to help the body increase insulin levels. This, in turn, lowers blood sugar.

If you follow a keto diet while taking these medications, it might cause you to develop hypoglycemia. It is very important to talk to your doctor so you can work together to prevent the risk of developing hypoglycemia before you start a keto diet.

Testing your blood sugar allows you to spot and possibly avoid developing hypoglycemia. You are going to have to test more often than normal while you are getting used to the changes in the intake of carbs.

Blood Sugar Issues or Diabetes

Some people that try the keto diet will have problems with some low blood sugar or hypoglycemia at the beginning. This could be dangerous if you can't get your blood sugar stabilized while taking your diabetes medications.

There is evidence that shows diabetes can be prevented or slowed down with a healthy diet and exercise. To keep you safe, if you have a history of prediabetes, diabetes, or hypoglycemia, you shouldn't try the keto diet without talking to your doctor first.

With the changes to your diet and any weight might mean the dosage of your diabetes medication might need to be adjusted. You shouldn't follow any type of restrictive diet without being supervised by your doctor.

Other Medicines

Other medications shouldn't cause any major risks but might need to be looked at to make sure you are still in need of it. Your doctor will be able to tell you if any changes are needed.

Blood pressure medicines might need to be regulated by your doctor, since your blood pressure might go down while on a keto diet.

Nutrient Deficient or Underweight

Even though the keto diet is a high-fat diet, it could lead to weight loss and this might happen very quickly. If you are already underweight, have any mineral or vitamin deficiencies because you aren't eating enough, or have had any eating disorders in the past, you should not do this diet.

If you have a low BMI and want to try the keto diet to help improve your blood sugar level but aren't looking to lose weight, you absolutely must talk to your doctor or a dietitian before you start this diet. They can help you modify the diet to make sure your weight won't be affected.

If you can lose weight easily, a diet that includes complex carbs along with a lot of healthy fats and proteins might be a better fit for you.

If you have undergone gastric bypass surgery, this diet could be extremely dangerous for you since the risk of nutrient deficiencies might happen from not consuming enough calories.

Gall Bladder Removal or Gallstones

People that have had gallstones were told to stay away from fat but this isn't true now. The NHS says that low-fat diets could actually cause gallstones to grow.

If you have gallstones now, eating more fat might cause you some pain. If you want to try the keto diet, you may need to go very slow or try the diet after your gallstones have been removed or dissolved.

A study done in 2014 showed that high-fat diets might actually prevent gallstones from forming which may be a long-term benefit of the keto diet.

Even though the gallbladder has bile in it that helps to break down fats, it has been reported that by following a high-fat, low-carb diet without having a gallbladder can be successful.

Many people without gall bladders have been very successful on the keto diet without reporting any adverse side effects.

Kidney Stones or Kidney Disease

Kidney stones are a side effect that has been caused by the keto diet. If you have a history of kidney disease, it probably isn't worth the risk of trying the keto diet.

If you have a family history of any kind of kidney disease, you must talk with your doctor before beginning the keto diet. Your doctor will need to check your creatinine/calcium ratio to make sure you aren't risking any complications such as nephrolithiasis which is a dangerous level of calcium in the kidneys.

Children

The keto diet has been used for many years in children who have seizures to help keep them under control. This must be done under the supervision of a doctor.

There are some things to keep in mind before starting a keto diet to make sure all the macronutrients are balanced and appropriate for children.

You absolutely must consult your doctor or dietitian before beginning keto diet on any child.

Enzyme Deficiency or Defect

These disorders are extremely rare, but there are two serious contraindications of the keto diet called porphyria and pyruvate carboxylase deficiency. These conditions are caused by problems with the production of heme and lipid metabolism. Heme is found in hemoglobin that carries oxygen out of the lungs and into other parts of the body.

People that have these disorders will have deficiencies with certain enzymes that will make it hard to metabolize large amounts of free fatty acids. They will then transport them to the cell's mitochondria to create energy. If you are on the keto diet and have these deficiencies or other types of beta oxidations defects, it could cause extremely dangerous complications like mental changes, irregular heartbeats, and nervous system deterioration.

Free fatty acids get built up in the body and can't be used for energy. This is the main reason it is dangerous. People who have porphyria and pyruvate carboxylase deficiency need a steady supply of glucose to give their organs energy. If there isn't any glucose present due to the keto diet, some life-threatening problems might happen. This is called a catabolic crisis. To stay away from these complications, if you have a family history of mitochondrial disorders or suspect you might have any of these conditions, you must be tested by your doctor before you even think about going on the keto diet.

Exercise

Everyone knows that when you exercise, you are going to have better health. When you follow a keto diet, you are going to lose weight fast and improve your health. What would happen if you combined the two?

It would be reasonable to assume, if you combined the two it would take your weight loss and health to another level. The truth is a bit more complicated. With being restricted on your intake of carbs, there is a huge amount of change that is going to happen, and some of these are going to affect your exercise.

With the restrictive intake of carbs, you are limiting your muscle cells from getting glucose, which has always been the easiest fuel source. When our muscles can't access glucose, their high-intensity function is impaired. High intensity stands for any activity that lasts longer than ten seconds. The reason for this is that after ten seconds of maximum effort, the muscles begin turning to glucose for energy through a metabolic pathway known as glycolysis instead of the phosaphen system.

Fat and ketones aren't a good substitute for glucose during this time. Only after you have been exercising for two minutes will your body shift into this metabolic pathway that will use your fat and ketones.

Basically, when you restrict your intake of carbs, you deprive the cells in your muscles of glucose, which they need for fuel during the high-intensity effort for ten seconds to two minutes. This just means that if you are doing a ketogenic diet, it is going to limit your performance during exercises such as:

- Swimming or sprinting for more than ten seconds.
- Weightlifting for more than five reps each set using a weight that is heavy enough to bring you close to failure.
- High-intensity circuit training or interval training.
- Playing a sport that gives you minimal breaks like soccer, lacrosse, and rugby.

This list isn't a comprehensive one, but it gives you a good idea of the types of exercises that your body uses glycolysis for. Remember though, that the metabolic pathway timing all depends on each individual person. There are some that can maintain performance for 30 seconds without needing any carbs.

It is also important that you eat the right amount of proteins and fats when you are exercising while following a keto diet.

Many health professionals, when designing a diet plan, will set the protein intake first. Protein gets the top priority because it performs many actions that fats and carbs can't. Protein helps to make you feel fuller longer, has a better thermic effect, and stimulates muscle synthesis better than any other macronutrients. If you don't eat enough protein, you might wind up losing muscle mass and consuming more calories than you need.

If you are going to keep your exercise regimen or begin one, which you really should, you need to make sure you eat the correct amount of macros. Here are some guidelines to follow.

- The biggest part of excess calories should come from healthy fats, not from carbs or protein.
- Keep your protein intake to a gram per pound of body weight.
- Be sure that your caloric intake stays around a deficit of 250 to 500 calories. This isn't of top priority. Many people won't worry about calories that much when doing a keto diet.

Now that we've established that you need to be smart and careful when eating while exercising, let's take a closer look at some specifics.

Keto and Cardio

Luckily for the majority of us, we aren't athletes so adding in an exercise routine isn't going to be that hard. Cardio workouts don't require you to exercise at high-intensities which require your body to burn glycogen and sugar for results. You just have to bring your heart rate up and keep it there.

Because cardio has a low to moderate intensity, a keto diet isn't going to impair your performance. You might even realize that you can workout longer without getting as tired when you are in ketosis.

The intensity you need to aim to get the most out of your workout is moderate intensity. When you are aiming for moderate-intensity physical activity, you should get your heart rate to about 50 to 70 percent of your maximum heart rate.

In order to estimate your maximum heart rate, begin by subtracting your age from 220. If you are a 50-year-old person, to figure out your age-related heart rate, you would take 220 and subtract 50. This gives you a total of 170 beats per minute. Then you could figure out the 50 to 70 percent levels, which will be:

- 70 percent – 170 x 0.70 = 119
- 50 percent – 170 x 0.50 = 85

This means a 50-year-old person, in order to partake in moderate-intensity physical activity needs to keep a heart rate between 85 and 119 beats per minute.

While your body is adapting to a ketogenic diet, you need to try to aim for the bottom end of that range. When you have been on the diet for a couple of weeks, you will begin to realize you can maintain a higher heart rate without needing extra carbs.

If you are new to working out and cardio, you want to stick to 50 percent of your maximum heart rate for about 10 to 15 minutes. You can begin to increase the duration by 5 or so each week until you are able to work out for 30 to 45 minutes at 50 percent of your maximum heart rate. When you have managed this, you can begin increasing your intensity level every week until you've reached 70 percent of your maximum heart rate.

If you aren't sure what works best for cardio workouts, here are a few examples.

- Interval training classes
- Aerobic training classes
- Cycling
- Swimming
- Recreational sports
- Circuit training
- Running

You need to remember though, that your power and strength could end up being decreased in these workouts because of carb restriction. If you are aiming for a good cardiovascular workout, then it isn't important that you push yourself to the max for your power and strength.

This isn't saying you can't increase your power and strength while doing a keto diet. All you have to do to achieve this is practice some mindful exercising.

Weight Lifting and Keto

You can increase muscle mass, power, and strength while following a keto diet. The best thing is that you can improve all of these things at the same time by using the same program.

Remember that I stated earlier that without glucose your body can only last for ten seconds when doing high-intensity exercises? This means that if you are a weightlifter, you can improve your power and strength, as well as muscle mass by doing sets that don't last longer than ten seconds.

This means that if you follow a program that requires five or more sets of five or fewer reps for each of the exercises, then this is perfect for people on a keto diet.

Some recent research has found that lower reps can be helpful when it comes to hypertrophy. This means that your muscles don't need you to pump out 8 to 12 reps in a row to grow bigger. What the muscles are looking for is the right amount of volume, which all depends on the individual person, and for your volume to increase every week.

This means that you are able to build muscles without carbs. Carbs might be needed for some high-intensity work, but a bodybuilder does not have to consume lots of carbs in order to see results.

Supplementing

There are a lot of no carb supplements out there that can help boosts your exercise performance while following a keto workout. Here are some keto friendly supplements.

1. Creatine

This is one of the most well-studied exercise supplement and it is an effective and safe way to enhance the body's phosphagen system. This is why creatine is best for explosive weightlifter and athletes.

Consuming five grams each day of creatine monohydrate powder is a great way to supplement for people who are looking to increase their muscle mass, power, and strength.

2. MCT or Medium Chain Triglycerides

MCTs as stated earlier are a form of saturated fats that get sent straight to the liver once they have been digested. The liver uses these fats for more ketones and is then sent to the cells that need the energy. MCTs are a great option for endurance athletes and cardio training.

It is recommended that you supplement with one or two tablespoons of MCT oil or powder before doing any endurance workouts to get an extra boost of energy

3. Exogenous ketones

These ketones, much like ketone esters and ketone salts, can provide you with an instant source of energy. There is a downside though. This supplement might end up lowering your liver's production of ketones, so it would be best if you used these with MCTs to boost ketone production.

A lot like MCTs, exogenous ketones are great for endurance and cardio training athletes. The main thing is to be sure you stay well hydrated when using these supplements because they do have a diuretic effect.

4. Caffeine

It isn't surprising that caffeine has been discovered as a great way to improve exercise performance because of its stimulatory effects. However, you could end up finding that you no longer get the same boost when you begin taking caffeine on a constant basis because of the way the body adapts to the habitual intake.

Plus caffeine might end up increasing your cortisol levels, which end up decreasing your ketone production. It is best if you experiment with the other supplements and limit the amount of caffeine you use.

5. Taurine

This is an organic acid that has been found to help exercise performance. In fact, researchers have discovered that it works better to help exercise performance than caffeine.

In a recent study, the scientists looked at the effects that taurine, caffeine and taurine, and caffeine had on fatigue and power on all-out cycling sprints. The taurine supplement that was used by itself was able to decrease fatigue and improve power than the other two supplements.

This has a big implication for bodybuilders and athletes who follow a keto diet because this study looked at the energy system that tends to be the most affected by carb restriction. According to the study, the participants took 50 mg of taurine per kilogram of weight. This would probably be a safe metric to use to figure out how much you need to take. You can also slowly decrease the amount to see if you still get any effects.

6. Fish oil

The omega 3 fatty acids, EPA, and DHA found in fish oil help to boost your recovery and stimulate muscle synthesis. The AHA recommends that you consume one gram of these each day. This can be reached through a fish oil supplement or by eating three ounces of salmon or sardines each day.

The goal of this is to help reduce your soreness. That means you need to aim for a six-gram dose that is spread throughout the day.

7. Protein Powder

While it is best for you to consume the majority of your protein from natural sources, protein powder is a good idea when you need help meeting your protein needs. This is also great if you follow a vegan keto diet.

You should make sure that you stick with complete protein powders such as collagen, whey, casein, or a mix of plant proteins. Stay away from BCAA and EAA supplements because you will receive better benefits from a complete protein powder.

Use this by adding 20 to 40 grams of protein powder to a smoothie or you could consume it after you work out to help stimulate muscle synthesis without affecting your ketosis.

8. Beta-alanine

This is a common compound in more pre-workout supplements that will give your body a tingly sensation. Most people report that they are able to perform one or two reps more when they are training in sets of eight to 15 when they take beta-alanine.

This means that this is probably a really good supplement for keto dieters that need a better glycolytic pathway to help them through their training. High-intensity athletes and bodybuilders will get the most from this supplement.

With this supplement, timing doesn't really matter. Aim for two to five grams of beta-alanine along with five grams of creatine each day. If you don't enjoy the tingly sensation that it gives you, you can take a gram of beta-alanine two to five times during the day.

9. Alpha GPC

Choline is an important part of your nervous system. Whenever you move a muscle in your body, choline is needed in order to activate acetylcholine, a neurotransmitter which will send a chemical signal to your muscles and will make them mobile. The best way to get more choline is through taking an alpha GPC supplement.

Research has found that 600 mg of it can help to enhance your power output and your secretion of growth hormones. This suggests that this choline supplement is great for weightlifters and athletes.

10. L-citrulline

This is a common supplement for cardiovascular health supplement and sports performance. Some studies have discovered that supplements of L-citrulline help to improve endurance and reduce fatigue for anaerobic and aerobic prolonged exercise. This is a great supplement for nearly every active person, except for those who rely on the phosphagensystem such as powerlifters and golfers. To help your exercise endurance, take 6,000 to 8,000 mg around an hour before you are going to work out.

Keto and Exercise in Harmony

To mix these two things, you have to make the right changes to your diet and workout program so that you don't cause any adverse reactions especially if you partake in high-intensity workouts.

When you are trying to add in exercise just to improve your health, then you can experiment with things a bit more than an athlete can. In general, you should try lifting weight and some cardio training every week. Cardio should be done two to three times each week and lift weights two to three times each week. You should avoid doing them both on the same day.

Keto While Vegan

Health, animal suffering, and climate change are three big issues that can be taken care of with a single solution, a vegan diet. At least, that's what a lot of health documentaries talk about. However, there is a more nuanced truth.

There are some that do better when they follow a low-carb diet with animal products, and then there are others that like a high-carb vegan diet. Following a vegan diet may not be the best diet for every health problem. For example, people that have epilepsy, Alzheimer's disease, Parkinson's disease, type 1 diabetes, type 2 diabetes, and obesity are helped tremendously when following a keto diet, while a vegan diet doesn't help them as much.

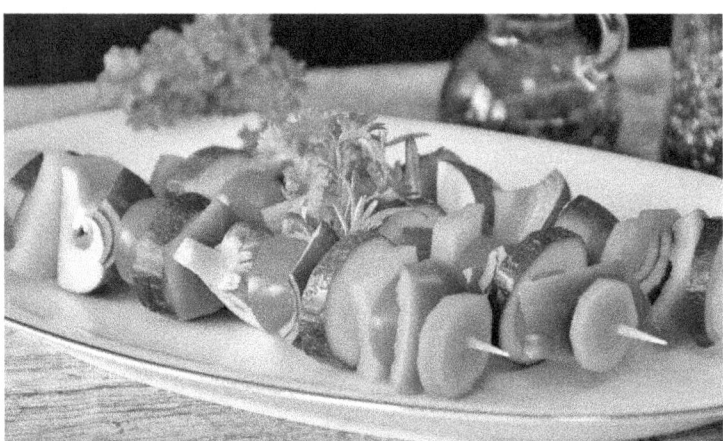

Now, does this mean that vegans need to give up their ethical concerns and start eating animal products? No. What should you do if you are following a high-carb vegan diet that isn't working for you and a keto diet could be exactly what you need, but it normally has too many animal products? Mix them.

An Overview

A vegan keto diet is an extremely restrictive diet, but you can pull it off and maintain your sanity, improve your health, and decrease animal suffering. In order to implement this correctly, follow these rules:

- Lower your carb intake to 35 grams or less.
- Get rid of all fish, meat, and other animal products.
- Consume plenty of veggies that are low in carbs.
- Make sure at least 70% of your calories are coming from plant-based fats.
- 25% of your calories need to come from plant-based proteins.
- Make sure you take supplements for your nutrients that you aren't getting from foods such as taurine, zinc, iron, EPA & DHA, B6, B12, and D3.

Limiting Carbs

It probably seems difficult enough to restrict the number of carbs you consume on a regular keto diet, so how is it going to go when you are following a vegan keto diet? Let's start out simply by looking at high-carb foods that you need to completely get rid of.

- Never Eat
    - Tubers like yams and potatoes.
    - Fruits like oranges, bananas, and apples.
    - Sugar like maple syrup, agave, and honey.
    - Legumes like peas, black beans, and lentils.
    - Grains like cereal, rice, corn, and wheat.

Now, the important part is finding vegan-friendly foods that are also low in carbs.

- Do Eat
    - Vegan protein like seitan, tofu, and tempeh.
    - Mushrooms like lion's mane, king oyster, and shiitake.
    - Leafy greens.
    - All above ground veggies like zucchini, cauliflower, and broccoli.
    - High-fat vegan dairy like vegan cheese, coconut cream, and coconut-based yogurt.

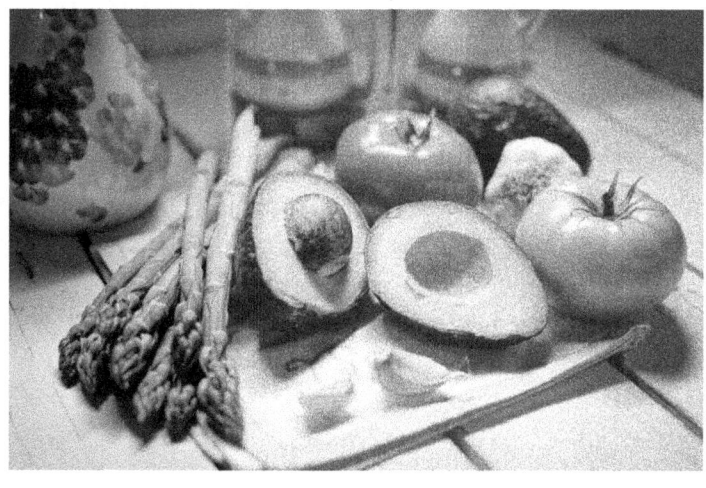

    - Seeds and nuts like pumpkin seeds, sunflower seeds, almonds, and pistachios.
    - Berries and avocado.
    - Fermented foods like kimchi, sauerkraut, and natto.
    - Sea vegetables like kelp, bladderwrack, dulse.
    - Sweeteners like monk fruit, erythritol, and stevia.
    - Other fats like avocado oil, MCT oil, olive oil, and coconut oil.

When you stick to the foods that are on the do eat list, you should be able to stick with a vegan keto diet and make sure that all of your nutritional bases are covered. At first though, you could find it difficult to adapt to this way of eating when many keto and low-carb recipes contain animal products. Luckily, all you have to do is make a couple of simple substitutions in order to veganize your keto recipes.

Simple Alternatives

If you buy a keto cookbook or search online for keto recipes, you are going to see a lot of recipes with cheese and eggs. There are also a lot of desserts full of high-fat dairy. That's where keto-friendly vegan substitutions come in.

- Substitute milk with coconut milk. The substitution works one to one, so if it calls for a cup of milk, use a cup of coconut milk.

- Substitute heavy cream with coconut cream. Depending on the creaminess of your coconut cream, you may find that you have to mix in some water or some of the water in the container.

- Replace butter with vegan butter or coconut oil. Coconut oil has a lower melting point but has the same smoke point as butter. This makes it a good replacement. If you don't like coconut oil, you can also use vegan butter. Check to make sure that there aren't any hydrogenated oils in the vegan butter because these increase your risk of heart disease.

- Instead of dairy cheese, use vegan cheese. There are a lot of vegan cheeses out there. If you don't want to use soy, then you can go for cashew, coconut, or other tree-nut cheeses.

- Replace cream cheese with vegan soft cheese. The company Treeline creates lots of cashew-based soft cheese and its texture is nearly identical to cream cheese. There are also ways to make your own cashew cheese.

- Instead of sour cream or yogurt, use nut-based yogurt. You can find coconut milk yogurts almost everywhere now and you may be able to find cashew or almond based yogurts. Check to make sure that there aren't any hidden sugars or carbs.

When you are purchasing keto-friendly vegan products, you need to check to make sure that they haven't added any sugars and that there aren't any hidden carbs or unhealthy ingredients such as hydrogenated oils. There are some products that use "gum" such as guar gum or agar agar. These are all compounds that are used to make them creamier and most people don't have a problem eating them. However, these products will cause gastrointestinal discomfort for some people, so check to see if your vegan dairy products have these added gums.

The great thing is that the availability of keto-friendly, dairy-free products have increased quickly. There are even some products that can be shipped straight to your home like Miyoko's Kitchen.

Now that we have looked at keto-friendly and vegan-friendly dairy choices, what to do about eggs? Eggs, egg yolks, and egg whites are important parts in a lot of delicious ketogenic recipes. As a vegan, do you need to ditch these?

Egg Substitutes

It can be so frustrating to find delicious but almost-vegan friendly recipes. You scroll through the list of ingredients and then you find it needs eggs. You don't have to fret just yet. You don't have to give up on these delicious foods. There are a lot of egg substitutes that you can use that are keto-friendly.

- Flax Seed

Ground up flax seeds makes a great binder. It tastes a bit nutty and works well in recipes that call for coconut or almond flour. Mix together a tablespoon of ground flax seeds with three tablespoons of water to replace an egg in a recipe.

- Silken Tofu

This is silkier and softer form of tofu that creates a great dairy and egg replacement. It's pretty much flavorless, but it may end up making your baked goods a bit dense, so it works best in brownies and some cakes and quick bread. A quarter of a cup of pureed silken tofu will replace an egg.

- Vinegar and baking soda

This is a good substitute for fluffier baked goods. A teaspoon of baking soda combined with a tablespoon of white vinegar will replace an egg.

If you don't want to make your own replacements, you can purchase ready-made vegan replacements.

- The Vegg

This company is 100% plant-based. They use only natural ingredients to create products that simulate the function, taste, and texture of eggs and it costs almost the same as real eggs.

- Follow Your Heart's VeganEgg

This is another plant-based company that makes vegan choices from mayo to cheese. That means they even have vegan eggs. Their VeganEgg is a whole egg replacement that has the texture and taste of actual eggs. These can be used to make cakes, muffins, and cookies. You can also scramble them up or use them to create omelets.

The main issue with these replacements is that they don't have the same protein or fat as a regular whole egg. This could make meeting all of your recommended macros on keto a little bit harder. Luckily, there are a lot of fats that you can eat from plant-based oils and lots of protein from vegan meat options.

Getting Enough Fat

While you aren't able to eat dairy, butter, meat, or eggs, you still have a lot of sources for fat on a vegan keto diet. Here are the best oils that you can have.

- Coconut oil

This is a great source of fat for baking, cooking, desserts, and fat bombs. It provides you with medium and long-chain saturated fatty acids that are a great source for fuel.

- Olive oil

This can be used to enhance the fat content and flavor a lot of dishes. Make sure that you keep temperatures under 405 degrees so that it doesn't end up oxidizing.

- Avocado oil

This oil has healthy monounsaturated fats than all of the other common oils. It also has the best smoke point at 520 degrees, which means it's great for deep frying, baking, and cooking.

- Red Palm oil

This is a great source of Vitamins A and E. It has a carrot-like flavor and buttery, rich texture. Its smoke point is a bit higher than coconut and olive oil. You do need to be careful when buying palm oil. There are a lot of palm oil products that are created in a way that hurts the wildlife, environment, and the workers that produce it.

That's why when you buy palm oil, look for bottles marked RSPO-certified or CSPO products. All of these companies produce products that are approved by the Roundtable on Sustainable Palm Oil. They use practices that meet strict social and environmental criteria. When you choose these products, you will be helping sustainable oil producers.

- MCT oil

This is often derived from palm and coconut oil. It is a medium chain triglyceride. These are saturated fatty acids that don't go through normal fat digestion and will head straight to your liver where it is changed into ketones. When you are looking for an energy boost, these can be added to hot drinks, fat bombs, sauces, and salads.

There are many other vegan oil options out there, but the ones listed provide you with health benefits and versatility. However, you aren't stuck with just oils to get your fat intake. You can find fat, as well as minerals and vitamins in these other foods: avocado, nuts, seeds, and vegan dairy substitutes.

With all of these fat-packed plant foods and oils, you shouldn't have a problem with getting the fats that you need on your vegan keto diet. The next thing you have to take care of, and probably the hardest, is getting your protein.

Vegan Protein Sources

Making sure that you get enough protein to maintain your health and muscle mass is hard enough for vegans, now you have to work with a keto diet. When you mix these diets, you are getting rid of a lot of amazing plant-based protein sources such as legumes.

When you can't have peas, lentils, and beans, how are you going to consume any protein?

Don't worry, there are other options.

- Tofu

This is a great substitute for all types of meats. Tofu is made from soybeans and contains lots of calcium and protein. While it does have a reputation of being blank, it has a great ability to absorb flavors from marinades and spices. If you make sure that you season your tofu before cooking it, it should taste delicious. You can also adjust the firmness and chewiness by purchasing extra-firm tofu and pressing out the water.

Since many vegan protein options contain soy, it's important to understand soy. Soy contains goitrogens, which can affect the thyroid. If you eat a lot of soy products and start experiencing unexplained weight gain, dry skin, constipation, cold sensitivity, and fatigue, you should limit your soy intake.

- Tempeh

This is a grainier and firmer tofu. This is made from fermented soybeans and is great to use for recipes calling for ground beef and fish. Tempeh doesn't have to be pressed like tofu, so only less step.

- Seitan

This is known as wheat meat and is made from seaweed, garlic, ginger, soy sauce, and wheat gluten. This is a great source of iron, low in fat and high in protein. If you are sensitive to gluten, you may want to avoid this protein source.

There are other "meat" sources that you can find in grocery stores. When you are trying to pick one out, make sure you read through the nutrition facts and ingredients. You don't want a product that has a lot of carbs or sugars. Try to find ones with the simplest ingredients and lowest carb content.

You can also turn to seeds and nuts to provide you with protein. They also contain important minerals and nutrients. Some good options are flaxseeds, sunflower seeds, almonds, pistachios, and pumpkin seeds. Make sure that you don't eat too many because they can rack up carbs.

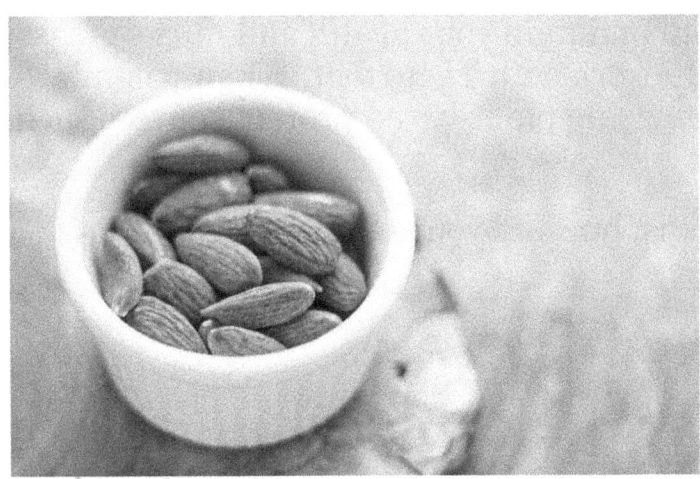

While peanuts are a legume, they are one of the only legumes that you can eat. They are low in carbs and high in protein.

The last vegan protein source is vegan protein powder. This is going to be your secret weapon. You can add flavorless vegan protein powders to your dishes to increase your protein content.

It is easier now to keep up with a vegan keto lifestyle. There are a lot of alternatives to dairy and eggs to help make veganizing your keto recipes easier. You shouldn't have any problems getting enough protein and fat in your diet. Make sure that you keep plenty of coconut oil, olive oil, various nuts, and seeds, as well as avocados on hand. Also, you should have vegan protein powder in your pantry.

Now, it's up to you to take control and start your vegan ketogenic diet.

FAQ

The majority of these questions have already been answered in the book but this section provides you with a quick reference guide to the most common questions that people have about the keto diet. If this doesn't give you enough in-depth answers, look for the chapter about your question.

Should I take supplements?

If you begin to feel a bit "crampy" or just don't feel like your normal self after you have begun a keto diet, you might want to look into certain supplements that will help you begin to feel better:

- o Vitamin B Complex
- o Multivitamins for Men
- o Potassium Supplement
- o Magnesium Supplement
- o Vitamin D Supplement
- o Multivitamins for Women

Always talk to your doctor before adding any supplements or vitamins to your diet.

Should I worry if I exercise?

There are usually two types of people that exercise. People that lift weights and people that run. If you do cardio exercises like running, biking, or participating in marathons, you really don't have to worry. Endurance training can be affected by the keto diet.

When lifting weights, you need to know what end results you want. Carbs could help your overall performance and help your muscles recover. By doing this, you will get better strength performance and faster gains when exercising. You can achieve this in a couple of ways, CKD and TKD.

CKD stands for the cyclical ketogenic diet and is a technique that is a bit more advanced. If you are just beginning keto, you don't need to do this. This is used more for competitors and bodybuilders. They used keto to help with building muscles while working out. To do this method, you do a normal keto diet for five days and then change to consuming more carbs for two days. By doing this, you will replenish all the glycogen stores in your body that will help you with the training that you do the other five days. Your goal is to get rid of all the stored glycogen.

TKD stands for the targeted ketogenic diet. With this technique, you eat carbs just before you workout to bump you out of ketosis when you exercise. It works by giving your muscles a needed supply of glycogen to use while working out. Once you have used up all this glycogen, your body will go back into ketosis.

My weight loss has stalled. What can I do?

Everybody on this planet who has ever attempted dieting has reached a weight loss plateau. There are a few things that might cause this to happen. There are many things that could help you over it. You could try fat fasting, intermittent fasting, change your eating habits, and cut out certain foods.

Here are some suggestions that might help you start losing weight again.

- Cut out processed foods
- Change to measuring yourself instead of weighing
- Stop consuming artificial sweeteners
- Lower the amount of carbs you consume
- Check all foods for hidden carbs
- Don't eat nuts
- Stop consuming dairy
- Increase your fat intake

What about alcohol?

You can drink alcohol while on a keto diet but you have to be careful. There are certain types of alcohol that do contain carbs.

If you absolutely have to drink, go for straight liquor. Don't drink cocktails, wine, or beer because these have carbs in them. Clear liquors are best. Just try to stay away from anything that is flavored. Those might have carbs in them.

I'm constipated. What can I do?

It is fairly normal for people who are just beginning the keto diet to start having irregular bowel movements. Here is a list of advice that can help with constipation or other bowel problems.

- Try eating flax or chia seeds
- Quit eating nuts (if you've been consuming a lot)
- Try drinking hot tea or coffee
- Try eating a tablespoon of coconut oil
- Eat more veggies that are high in fiber
- Try a magnesium supplement
- Drink more water

I'm feeling very bad. What do I need to do?

The most common problems for anyone who has started the keto diet are getting brain fogginess and headaches. When our bodies go into ketosis, we start urinating a lot more than normal and we lose a lot of water. Along with that, our bodies are burning up the fat it has stored over the years. This easily leads to disaster. When you urinate, you are expelling a lot of electrolytes from your body and you have to replace them.

Try to eat more salt and drink more water. Salty foods like bacon, deli meat, and salted are good to eat while the body is transitioning to ketosis. Drinking bone broth will also help increase the electrolytes in your body. These will help keep you functional and sane.

What are macros and do I need to count them?

Macros stand for macronutrients. The main macronutrients are carbohydrates, proteins, and fats. As we stated earlier, calories do matter and you must keep track of them when on this lifestyle. It gets you in the habit of watching them. It also lets you see how well you are doing. It's amazing just how much we will lie to ourselves about the number of carbs we put into our diet.

Keeping track of your macros can also help you if your weight loss stalls. You can easily see the things in your diet that could be causing your problem. When you are tracking macros, be sure you use grams and not percentages. Many people who are new to this diet think that just because their diet consists of 75 percent fat, 20 percent protein, and 5 percent carbs, they are doing well. This might not be the case. Grams give you a more accurate description of what you have eaten.

If you get off some of your macros, it isn't a huge deal. There is some wiggle room to go up or down by 10 to 15 grams of proteins or fats the majority of the time. If you happen to go over sometimes, or under sometimes, don't beat yourself up too much. If you keep your calories under control and they aren't in a deficit too far, you are going to be fine.

Could I have aheart attack from eating too much fat?

The three groups of fat you will be consuming are monounsaturated fats, polyunsaturated fats, and saturated fats. People use to think that saturated fats were bad for you because of a link between heart disease and saturated fats. In recent years, it has been proven that saturated fats do NOT cause heart attacks but can actually improve your cholesterol levels. You can eat saturated fats without worrying.

Polyunsaturated fats are a bit trickier. Processed polyunsaturated fats like vegetable oils and margarine spreads are very bad for you. These are loaded with trans fats. These do have a connection with heart disease and you should stay away from them at all costs. There are some polyunsaturated fats that are natural in some foods like fish that can actually improve cholesterol. You should try to find as many of these healthy fats as you can and stop eating the unhealthy ones.

Monounsaturated fats are known as healthy ones. Olive oil is the main example of an oil that is more of a monounsaturated fat than anything else. It is very healthy for us and could help lower your cholesterol.

How does ketosis work?

Ketosis happens when you don't consume carbohydrates. When you don't eat carbs, your body will begin consuming your stored body fat for the energy it needs. It is extremely healthy for you and it is great for your brain.

How does your body get energy from fat? When your body goes into ketosis, it lets your lever break down fats into ketones. These ketones give us the energy we need.

So, how does this add up to losing weight? When you have a caloric deficit, you aren't giving your body the energy it needs. Therefore, it has to dig into your stored fat to produce the energy it needs.

How to know if you are in ketosis?

Many people will use Ketostix to let them know when they get into ketosis. These can be found in most pharmacies. These are not very accurate. They generally let you know if you are or aren't in ketosis. If there is any purple or pink on the stick, this shows that your body is producing ketones. If the color is darker, it means you are dehydrated and your ketone levels are extremely concentrated.

Ketostix measures how much acetone is in the urine. These are also unused ketones. The ketone that your brain and body use for energy is called BHB or Beta-hydroxybutyrate. These are not measured by a Ketostix.

If you want results that are more accurate and reliable, you should use a blood ketone meter. These will show the correct amount of ketones that are in your blood. They don't get changed by hydration.

For more in-depth information, go back to the chapter on ketosis.

Will I lose alot of weight?

The amount of weight you will lose is totally up to you. As stated earlier, exercising is going to cause you to lose more weight. If you can completely stop eating foods that cause weight loss stalls like dairy, artificial sweeteners, and wheat products. Wheat products are anything that has any identifiable wheat product, wheat flours, and wheat gluten in it.

Losing water weight is normal when beginning a keto diet. Getting into ketosis has a diuretic effect on your body that helps you lose a large amount of weight in just a couple of days. Remember, you won't be losing fat right now, just water. This shows that your body is starting to turn itself into a machine to burn fat.

Am I consuming too much fat?

Yes, you could eat too much fat. The main point is you need to be in a caloric deficit to be able to lose weight. If you consume too much fat, it is going to push you over this deficit and will cause you to go into surplus that will cause you to gain weight. Most people can't overeat when on the keto diet since it is very low in carbs but high in fats, it is entirely possible.

Find a keto calculator to help you calculate your macros so you can see how many carbs, proteins, and fats you have to eat every day. Remember when you do this, you change the number of carbs and proteins you need according to your activity level.

Do I have to count calories?

Yes, calories do matter. The number of calories you consume and work off is an easy equation but it will never be true for everybody. Food sensitivities, endocrine disorders, and metabolic disorders all play a part in this. So what should you do? Eat right. Don't ever go into the deficit with calories and don't eat foods that are on the bad list.

When doing a keto diet, you usually don't have to worry about calories since the proteins and fats fill you up and keep you feeling fuller longer. If you like exercising, you need to take care and make sure your calories don't get into the deficit. Make sure you eat enough to make up for what you lost when you exercised.

How do I track my intake of carbs?

The easiest way to keep track of your intake of carbs is by using MyFitnessPal with their mobile app. This app won't let you track net carbs but you can track the total carbs you eat along with your total fiber. You could get net carbs by subtracting your fiber intake from the total carb intake. There are other apps out there like FatSecret that helps track the carb intake. Just do some research and find one that works for you.

Where can I find recipes?

Almost any health-conscious website will have recipes for you to look at. You can always just Google what you are craving and you will be amazed at the number of recipes that will pop up. You can take your favorite recipe and convert them into low carb just by getting rid of the sugars and fruit in them. Instead of using sugar just substitute it for artificial sweeteners.

How quickly will I get into ketosis?

A keto diet isn't one that you can just pick and choose when you are going to do it. Your body has to adjust to the diet before it gets into ketosis and this will take time. This can take anywhere from two to seven days. It all depends on what you eat, your activity level, and your body type. The quickest way to get your body into ketosis is learning to exercise before you eat anything. Keep your carb intake to less than 20 grams each day. Remember to drink plenty of water.

Myths

The keto diet is all the rage now and you've probably heard a lot about it. You haven't tried it yet because you have heard all sorts of rumors. Let's talk about some of the most famous myths going around about the keto diet.

Everyone isn't going to get the keto flue and everyone's body is different and will react differently to this diet. Factors like your age, gender, overall health, and activity level will affect your metabolism, how healthy your hormones are, and how your body will adapt to ketosis. Let's look at these myths and find the truth behind them.

Keto is a high-protein, high-fat diet

The keto diet isn't like other low-carb diets or the Atkins Diet. It isn't high in protein. The intake of protein needs to be moderate because this helps your body get into ketosis and helps it say there. Eating too much protein is going to cause it to be changed into glucose. This won't help keep your glucose at low levels.

You are probably wondering just how much protein you need to consume. Normally, you need to get about 20 percent of your daily calories from protein, five percent needs to come from carbohydrates, and 75 percent will come from fat, where a low-carb, high-protein diet requires you to eat around 30 to 35 percent of your daily calories from protein.

You will just lose weight on this diet

This diet helps people lose weight and burn stored fat from their bodies. Even if you don't want to lose weight, you can still do this diet to maintain your weight. It can actually help you gain some weight.

Yes, you read that right. You can gain some weight while doing this diet. It is possible if you don't do it the correct way and your body doesn't get into ketosis.

There is a lot of controversy about diets that are low in carbs and high in fat because most people think you can only lose weight if you have a low-calorie intake. Others believe it is due to changes in the hormones that this diet causes. Most experts agree that the diet actually doesn't matter. If the calories you eat exceed the amount of activity you do, you are going to gain weight instead of losing it.

If you eat more calories than what your body needs, even if they are from healthy fats and protein, you are going to see an increase in the number on your scale.

If you don't want to lose weight, should you do this diet? There are numerous benefits of the keto diet that go beyond weight loss. This diet will help your body normalize blood sugar, improve digestive health, regulate hormone production, improve cognitive function, and could actually reduce the risk of getting heart disease or diabetes.

There's noscience behind this diet

This is so false, it's hilarious. As stated earlier, this diet could help manage health problems such as Alzheimer's disease, cancer, epilepsy, muscle loss, high blood pressure, type 2 diabetes, dyslipidemia, obesity, and insulin resistance.

Can't exercise when doing keto

Exercising helps everybody, including people who are doing the keto diet. You may not feel energized when your body is transitioning into ketosis but this will lessen as your body adjusted to it. Even when you do high-intensity workouts, this diet won't cause any decline to your performance.

You don't have to stop working out when doing this diet. You may have to change up some of your workouts. If your body can handle it, exercising when you are in ketosis will help your body burn fat two to three times faster. This can help you maintain blood glucose levels. You might even notice you don't feel as fatigued.

To ensure you help your body while working out, make sure you eat enough calories especially those from fats. You need to let your body recover in between hard workouts.

If you are struggling while working out and you have a hard time recovering, try to eat more carbs right before you exercise. If you like to fast while doing the keto diet, save the high-intensity workout for when you have eaten more fuel.

You will lose muscle

This is another very false rumor. On the keto diet, you can actually gain muscle mass. If you can combine the keto diet with strength training, you could build muscle and increase your strength. The American Heart Association claims that these types of diets will cause a loss in muscle tissue. I don't know where they got that from but there are not any physiological requirements that humans have to eat carbs. This diet will not cause anyone to lose muscle mass.

Will this diet work if you don't exercise? Yes! It could lead to many improvements in your overall health. Exercising will kick things into high gear when talking about health benefits and body composition.

Everyone gets the keto flu

Every person is going to react differently to the keto diet. This makes it difficult to find out what side effects you are going to experience, how bad the effects are going to be, and how long they will last. Some people are going to transition into ketosis smoothly. Other may develop brain fog, sleep problems, more fatigue, and digestive problems for several weeks after getting into ketosis.

These side effects can be uncomfortable but they will go away in a week or so. You just have to be patient. You could lessen these by drinking more water, eating more fiber and salt, and getting more electrolytes from vegetables.

You won't have any energy doing keto

Many people say the energy and concentration increased after their body adjusted into ketosis. Your energy might be a bit lower when beginning this diet. After your body begins making ketones, it will give your brain a steady source of fuel. You might realize you are having better moods, the focus has increased, and you have more mental clarity after your body has become accustomed to the keto diet.

Remain on the diet for short periods of time

When you first begin the keto diet, you should just stay on this diet for two to three months and take a break. You have to give your body three weeks to get adjusted and then start back on the keto diet. If your body adjusts quickly to this, you can continue doing this for months and possibly years. Just listen to your body.

You can cheat on the keto diet

It really isn't realistic to remain on this diet for eternity. Cheat days are encouraged on other diets to give some support to your metabolism and to give you a break. When you cheat on the keto diet, it could bring you out of ketosis.

This may not be a problem if you do it intentionally. If you are aware of what is happening and can adjust your diet, coming out of ketosis is fine every now and then. If you realize you are no longer in ketosis since you have been cheating and consuming more carbs, take a few days to get back into eating right and cut back on the carbs.

You can eat any fat on keto just like with Atkins

Yes. Most of the calories on this diet come from fat. This isn't giving you permission to consume every saturated fat out there. Because keto isn't about just losing weight, you can eat healthy fats. Atkins lets you eat any fatty foods. Most people who try the keto diet want you to stay away from processed meats like bacon, salami, and sausage.

You are able to eat clean and avoid cheeses, poor quality meats, fried foods, processed foods, fast food, and trans fats if you want to get the most out of this diet. If you want to eat healthier, choose cage-free, organic eggs, pasture raised poultry, wild caught fish, avocados, nuts, grass-fed butter, grass-fed meats, and cold pressed oils like extra virgin olive oil or coconut oil.

Women and men are exactly the same withketo

Women are normally a bit more sensitive to dietary changes and weight loss than men. It might be possible for women to follow this diet and stay safe. They could also incorporate intermittent fasting if wanted. Women have to be sure they consume more non-starchy veggies to replenish their electrolytes and nutrients.

Women need to try to reduce the amount of stress that is in their lives and listen to their bodies. Stress can cause hormonal changes that can keep them out of ketosis. Pay attention to what your body is telling you when you workout. Exercise will impact your mood, your energy, how well you sleep, how much alcohol and caffeine you consume, how long you are out in the sun, and how many environmental toxins you are exposed to. If you start feeling run down or overwhelmed, you have to adjust your diet accordingly. If you push your body too hard, it might fight back.

You have to fast when doing keto

Fasting while on the keto diet isn't a requirement. You can choose whether or not you want to fast. You shouldn't fast until your body has adjusted into ketosis. After your body is used to consuming lower cabs, introducing intermittent fasting might have several benefits for your body. It could help with cravings, controlling hunger, speeding up weight loss, and detoxifying your body.

Some think that fasting is hard since you will feel hungry but this isn't true. If you eat the right amounts of veggies, protein, and fats, you are going to feel fuller longer. Fasting isn't as challenging as most people think it is.

No alcohol

Cocktails, beer, and wine are full of carbs. If you must have alcohol, there are options for you while doing the keto diet. Many liquors, light beers, and dry wines are very low in carbs.

You don't have to totally give up alcohol. You just need to be more conscious of what you are choosing. You need to also be careful when drinking because your body isn't full of carbs that absorb the alcohol. You might not be as tolerable to alcohol as you used to be. If you do drink, make sure you drink while you are eating since the fat and protein helps your body absorb the alcohol and prevents surges in blood sugar.

It's dangerous

Just like any diet or lifestyle change, there will be downsides but this diet isn't dangerous.

There are potential problems such as increased cholesterol and heart disease, gastrointestinal distress, decreased bone density, mineral and vitamin deficiencies, and kidney stones. These can be helped and avoided by adding supplements to your diet.

You absolutely have to keep yourself hydrated and go slowly into fasting if you have decided to. Be sure you know what your daily macros need to be and be sure you are hitting them. If you do all this, you will probably avoid all these problems.

Final thoughts

In spite of everything you have probably heard about the keto diet, it is relatively safe for most people to do for a long time. It could help you build muscles if you add in strength training. You might increase your energy levels due to your body burning more fat.

Most people think you only lose weight when doing the keto diet. The keto diet creates low energy and many other problems. Many think it is not safe for women to do for any amount of time since it could cause loss of muscle mass.

The keto diet is low in carbs and high in fats that will change the way the body burns fat for energy. It will stop burning sugar and carbs we eat and begin burning the fat that is stored in the body.

Good Foods

Now that you have all the information about the keto diet, let's find out exactly what you will be able to eat while on this new lifestyle. You will also get a list of what foods you need to avoid.

What to Eat

- Meats – all meats that are unprocessed are low in carbs and great for your new lifestyle. The best for you are ones that are organic, grass-fed meats. You need to remember that you are eating more fats than protein, so don't go crazy with meats. Look out for processed meats such as sausages, cold cuts, and meatballs. They will sometimes contain added carbs.

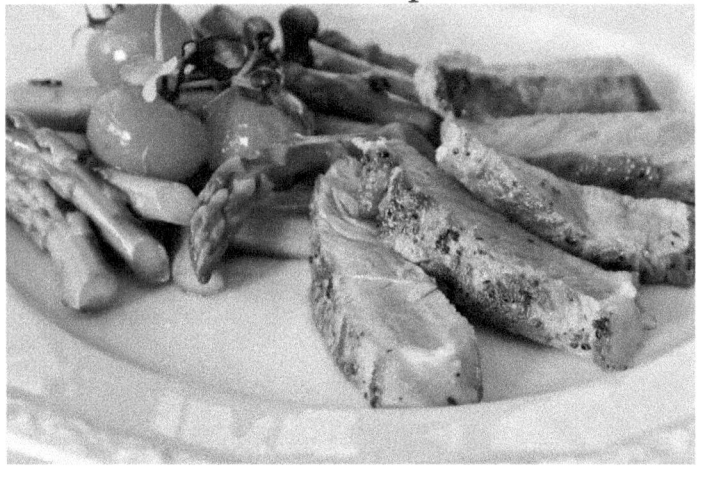

- Seafood and fish – all fish are good options, especially salmon. Salmon is high in Omega 3 fatty acids which our bodies need.

- Eggs – these are the most versatile foods you can eat on this diet because they can be fixed in so many different ways.

- High-fat sauces – most of the fats you consume needs to come from sources such as meat, fish, and eggs. You can also use butter and coconut oil to cook with to add fats into your diet.

- Vegetables that grow above ground – choose vegetables that grow above ground like green vegetables. The best ones are:
    - Zucchini
    - Avocado
    - Kale
    - Cauliflower
    - Brussels sprouts
    - Cabbage
    - Green beans

- o Broccoli
- o Asparagus
- o Spinach

- Dairy that is high in fat – the more fat it has in it, the better it is for this diet. Butter is the best. Make sure to get real butter and not margarine. Cheese that is high in fat is also great. High-fat yogurts need to be eaten in moderation. Normal milk is high in sugars so you need to stay away from it.

- Nuts – you can eat these in moderation. The best ones are Brazil, macadamia, and pecans.

- Berries – these can also be eaten in moderation. These include strawberries, blackberries, raspberries, and blueberries.

- Water – you absolutely have to drink a lot of water.

- Coffee – this is fine as long as you don't add anything to it except coconut oil and butter.

- Tea – this is also fine as long as you don't add sugar to it.

- Bone broth – consuming this can help add nutrients and electrolytes back into the diet.

- Alcohol – if you absolutely have to drink any alcohol, you can drink brandy, whiskey, vodka, and dry wine. Just make sure you don't consume anything that has added sugar.

- Dark chocolate – you need to find chocolate that has more than 70 percent cocoa in it. 85 percent is the ideal amount.

Foods to Avoid

- Sugar – this is a huge no-no. You absolutely have to stay away from soft drinks, fruit juices, vitamin water, and sports drinks. You also have to stay away from these:
    - o Donuts

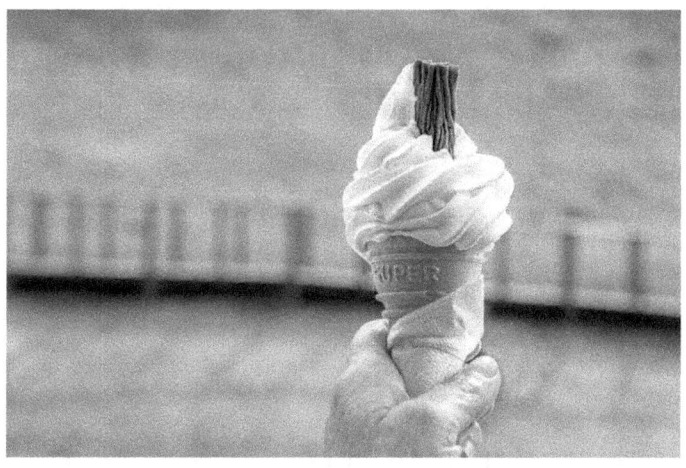

- o Breakfast cereals
- o Sweets

- - Frozen treats
  - Candy
  - Chocolate bars
  - Cakes
  - Cookies
- Starches
  - Sweet potatoes
  - Porridge
  - Muesli
  - Bread
  - Rice
  - Potato chips
  - Pasta
  - French fries
  - Beans
  - Potatoes
  - Lentils
- Beer – this is nothing more than liquid bread.
- Fruits
- Pre-packaged low-carb foods – these are not necessarily good for you. Be sure to read the label before you purchase these. Most of the Atkins products are not really low in carbs.
- Margarine – you have to use real butter. Never ever eat margarine, it is so bad for you.

Shopping List

In order to get you started on this diet the right way, this chapter is going to give you a shopping list that will help you get everything you are going to need. It has been organized by the types of food in order to help with your travels in the grocery store.

- **Vegetables**
    - Zucchini
    - Summer squash
    - Spaghetti squash
    - Sprouts
    - Garlic
    - Onions
    - Lettuce
    - Cucumbers
    - Bell pepper
    - Cabbage
    - Cauliflower
    - Broccoli
- **Fruits**
    - Strawberries
    - Raspberries
    - Blackberries
    - Blueberries
    - Avocados
- **Seafood**
    - Trout
    - Tuna
    - Shrimp
    - Salmon
- **Meats**
    - Pepperoni
    - Luncheon meats – make sure you read the label to see if they have added nitrites or carbs

- Hotdogs
- Bratwurst
- Elk
- Buffalo
- Venison
- Ground lamb
- Lamb Chops
- Pork steaks
- Ham steaks
- Ground Pork
- Pork ribs
- Polish sausage
- Kielbasa
- Bacon
- Breakfast sausage
- Duck
- Whole chicken
- Chicken breast
- Chicken thighs
- Ribeye steak
- Chuck roast
- Ground beef 80/20

- **Dairy**
  - Greek yogurt
  - Hard cheeses
  - Butter
  - Sour cream

- Eggs
- Cream cheese
- Heavy cream

- **Fats and oils**
  - Sesame oil
  - Coconut oil
  - Grapeseed oil
  - Olive oil
  - Avocado oil

- **Miscellaneous**
  - Pork rinds
  - Olives
  - Beef jerky
  - Full-fat ranch dressing
  - Sugar-free salad dressings
  - Salsa
  - Hot sauce
  - Cider vinegar
  - Mustard
  - Pickle juice
  - Sugar-free pickles
  - Chicken stock
  - No-sugar-added sauces
  - Nut Flours
  - Seeds
  - Nuts
  - Almond butter

- Sunflower butter
- Peanut butter

30-Day Meal Plan

So that you can get started, here is your 30-day meal plan. Before you start, make sure that you know all of your macro numbers.

Day 1

Breakfast: Two eggs and two slices of bacon – 1 gram net carb

Lunch: An avocado with pork rinds – 2 grams net carb

Dinner: Tuna salad with two hard boiled eggs, bibb lettuce, a half cup of almonds, an apple, and a cucumber – 13 grams net carb

Day 2

Breakfast: Bulletproof coffee – 0-gram net carb

Lunch: Serving of sunflower seeds – 4 grams net carbs

Dinner: Two ounces of turkey breast, hard-boiled egg, a quarter cup of cherry tomatoes, an ounce of sharp cheddar, four pita bites, two tablespoons almonds – 13 grams net carbs

Day 3

Breakfast: One boiled egg with a tablespoon mayo – 1 gram net carb

Lunch: 1/3 cup of hummus with pork rinds – 9 grams of net carb

Dinner: Chicken salad with balsamic vinegar dressing – 6 grams net carb

Day 4

Breakfast: Romaine lettuce leaf with a half ounce of butter, an ounce of cheese, half avocado, and a cherry tomato – 3 grams net carb

Lunch: String cheese – 1 gram of net carb

Dinner: Two ounces of turkey breast, hard-boiled egg, a quarter cup of cherry tomatoes, an ounce of sharp cheddar, four pita bites, two tablespoons almonds – 13 grams net carbs

Day 5

Breakfast: Two scrambled eggs – 1 gram net carb

Lunch: 1/3 cup of hummus with pork rinds – 9 grams of net carb

Dinner: Chicken salad with balsamic vinegar dressing – 6 grams net carb

Day 6

Breakfast: Two scrambled eggs with an avocado and two ounces of smoked salmon – 5 grams net carb

Lunch: Full-fat laughing cow cheese – 1 gram net carb

Dinner: Tuna salad with two hard boiled eggs, bibb lettuce, a half cup of almonds, an apple, and a cucumber – 13 grams net carb

Day 7

Breakfast: Two fried eggs – 1 gram net carb

Lunch: 1/3 cup of hummus with pork rinds – 9 grams of net carb

Dinner: Chicken salad with balsamic vinegar dressing – 6 grams net carb

Day 8

Breakfast: Two hardboiled eggs mashed into three ounces of butter – 1 gram net carb

Lunch: Quest bar – 5 grams net carb

Dinner: Two ounces of turkey breast, hard-boiled egg, a quarter cup of cherry tomatoes, an ounce of sharp cheddar, four pita bites, two tablespoons almonds – 13 grams net carbs

Day 9

Breakfast: An avocado with three ounces of deli turkey, an ounce of lettuce, and an ounce and a half of cream cheese – 9 grams net carb

Lunch: Serving of pork rinds – 0 grams net carb

Dinner: Chicken salad with balsamic vinegar dressing – 6 grams net carb

Day 10

Breakfast: An avocado fill with a third of a cup of mayo and three ounces of smoked salmon – 6 grams net carb

Lunch: Full-fat laughing cow cheese – 1 gram net carb

Dinner: Roll three slices of cheese in three slices of turkey and serve with a half of an avocado, cucumber slices, blueberries, and almonds – 13 grams net carb

Day 11

Breakfast: A cup of coffee with four tablespoons heavy cream – 2 grams net carb

Lunch: An avocado with pork rinds – 2 grams net carb

Dinner: Tuna salad with two hardboiled eggs, bibb lettuce, a half cup of almonds, an apple, and a cucumber – 13 grams net carb

Day 12

Breakfast: Two eggs and two slices of bacon – 1 gram net carb

Lunch: Quest bar – 5 grams net carb

Dinner: Two ounces of turkey breast, hard-boiled egg, a quarter cup of cherry tomatoes, an ounce of sharp cheddar, four pita bites, two tablespoons almonds – 13 grams net carbs

Day 13

Breakfast: Two fried eggs – 1 gram net carb

Lunch: 1/3 cup of hummus with pork rinds – 9 grams of net carb

Dinner: Chicken salad with balsamic vinegar dressing – 6 grams net carb

Day 14

Breakfast: Two hardboiled eggs mashed into three ounces of butter – 1 gram net carb

Lunch: An avocado with pork rinds – 2 grams net carb

Dinner: Tuna salad with two hardboiled eggs, bibb lettuce, a half cup of almonds, an apple, and a cucumber – 13 grams net carb

Day 15

Breakfast: Bulletproof coffee – 0-gram net carb

Lunch: Serving of sunflower seeds – 4 grams net carbs

Dinner: Two ounces of turkey breast, hardboiled egg, a quarter cup of cherry tomatoes, an ounce of sharp cheddar, four pita bites, two tablespoons almonds – 13 grams net carbs

Day 16

Breakfast: An avocado with three ounces of deli turkey, an ounce of lettuce, and an ounce and a half of cream cheese – 9 grams net carb

Lunch: Serving of pork rinds – 0 grams net carb

Dinner: Roll three slices of cheese in three slices of turkey and serve with a half avocado, cucumber slices, blueberries, and almonds – 13 grams net carb

Day 17

Breakfast: One boiled egg with a tablespoon mayo – 1 gram net carb

Lunch: 1/3 cup of hummus with pork rinds – 9 grams of net carb

Dinner: Chicken salad with balsamic vinegar dressing – 6 grams net carb

Day 18

Breakfast: A cup of coffee with four tablespoons of heavy cream – 2 grams net carb

Lunch: An avocado with pork rinds – 2 grams net carb

Dinner: Tuna salad with two hard boiled eggs, bibb lettuce, a half cup of almonds, an apple, and a cucumber – 13 grams net carb

Day 19

Breakfast: Romaine lettuce leaf with a half ounce of butter, an ounce of cheese, half avocado, and a cherry tomato – 3 grams net carb

Lunch: String cheese – 1 gram of net carb

Dinner: Two ounces of turkey breast, hard-boiled egg, a quarter cup of cherry tomatoes, an ounce of sharp cheddar, four pita bites, two tablespoons almonds – 13 grams net carbs

Day 20

Breakfast: Two scrambled eggs – 1 gram net carb

Lunch: 1/3 cup of hummus with pork rinds – 9 grams of net carb

Dinner: Chicken salad with balsamic vinegar dressing – 6 grams net carb

Day 21

Breakfast: An avocado fill with a third of a cup of mayo and three ounces of smoked salmon – 6 grams net carb

Lunch: Full-fat laughing cow cheese – 1 gram net carb

Dinner: Roll three slices of cheese in three slices of turkey and serve with a half avocado, cucumber slices, blueberries, and almonds – 13 grams net carb

Day 22

Breakfast: An avocado with three ounces of deli turkey, an ounce of lettuce, and an ounce and a half of cream cheese – 9 grams net carb

Lunch: Serving of pork rinds – 0 grams net carb

Dinner: Chicken salad with balsamic vinegar dressing – 6 grams net carb

Day 23

Breakfast: Two hard boiled eggs mashed into three ounces of butter – 1 gram net carb

Lunch: Quest bar – 5 grams net carb

Dinner: Roll three slices of cheese in three slices of turkey and serve with a half avocado, cucumber slices, blueberries, and almonds – 13 grams net carb

Day 24

Breakfast: A cup of coffee with four tablespoons of heavy cream – 2 grams net carb

Lunch: An avocado with pork rinds – 2 grams net carb

Dinner: Two ounces of turkey breast, hard-boiled egg, a quarter cup of cherry tomatoes, an ounce of sharp cheddar, four pita bites, two tablespoons almonds – 13 grams net carbs

Day 25

Breakfast: Two fried eggs – 1 gram net carb

Lunch: 1/3 cup of hummus with pork rinds – 9 grams of net carb

Dinner: Chicken salad with balsamic vinegar dressing – 6 grams net carb

Day 26

Breakfast: Two eggs and two slices of bacon – 1 gram net carb

Lunch: An avocado with pork rinds – 2 grams net carb

Dinner: Tuna salad with two hard boiled eggs, bibb lettuce, a half cup of almonds, an apple, and a cucumber – 13 grams net carb

Day 27

Breakfast: An avocado with three ounces of deli turkey, an ounce of lettuce, and an ounce and a half of cream cheese – 9 grams net carb

Lunch: Serving of pork rinds – 0 grams net carb

Dinner: Chicken salad with balsamic vinegar dressing – 6 grams net carb

Day 28

Breakfast: Romaine lettuce leaf with a half ounce of butter, an ounce of cheese, half avocado, and a cherry tomato – 3 grams net carb

Lunch: String cheese – 1 gram of net carb

Dinner: Tuna salad with two hard boiled eggs, bibb lettuce, a half cup of almonds, an apple, and a cucumber – 13 grams net carb

Day 29

Breakfast: Bulletproof coffee – 0-gram net carb

Lunch: Serving of sunflower seeds – 4 grams net carbs

Dinner: Two ounces of turkey breast, hard-boiled egg, a quarter cup of cherry tomatoes, an ounce of sharp cheddar, four pita bites, two tablespoons almonds – 13 grams net carbs

Day 30

Breakfast: Two fried eggs – 1 gram net carb

Lunch: 1/3 cup of hummus with pork rinds – 9 grams of net carb

Dinner: Chicken salad with balsamic vinegar dressing – 6 grams net carb

Conclusion

Thank you for making it through the end of *The Ketogenic Diet for Beginners*. Let's hope it was informative and able to provide you with all of the tools you need to achieve your goals whatever they may be.

Losing weight has always been a struggle, but with the keto diet, it becomes easier. Use the information found in this book to help get you started on a ketogenic diet.

Finally, if you found this book useful in anyway, a review on Amazon is always appreciated!

www.ingramcontent.com/pod-product-compliance
Lightning Source LLC
Chambersburg PA
CBHW080214040426
42333CB00044B/2677